Tertiary Care - Medical, Psychosocial, and Environmental Aspects

Edited by Ayşe Emel Önal

Published in London, United Kingdom

Tertiary Care - Medical, Psychosocial, and Environmental Aspects
http://dx.doi.org/10.5772/intechopen.110957
Edited by Ayşe Emel Önal

Contributors
Somprakas Basu, Navin Kumar, Aakansha Giri Goswami, Dhiraj Mallik, Sudhir Kumar Singh, Farhanul Huda, Adekunle Olowe, Olawumi Otutu, Rita Ayanbolade Olowe, Lucy Matsayi Aji, Ahmad Baba Muhammad, Hassan Abubakar, Nour Hanah Othman, Aina Amanina Abdul Jalil, Syarifah Syamimi Putri Adiba Syed Putera, Nor Safwan Hadi Nor Afendi, Sailaja Kallakuri, Buddha P.V., Mbulaheni Rhona Luphai, Ahmed Darwish, Malika Taufiq, Maliha Taufiq, Filippo Marino, Francesco Rossi, Emilio Sacco

First published in London, United Kingdom, 2024 by IntechOpen
IntechOpen is the global imprint of INTECHOPEN LIMITED, registered in England and Wales, registration number: 11086078, 5 Princes Gate Court, London, SW7 2QJ, United Kingdom

British Library Cataloguing-in-Publication Data
A catalogue record for this book is available from the British Library

Additional hard and PDF copies can be obtained from orders@intechopen.com

Tertiary Care - Medical, Psychosocial, and Environmental Aspects
Edited by Ayşe Emel Önal
p. cm.
Print ISBN 978-1-83769-138-8
Online ISBN 978-1-83769-139-5
eBook (PDF) ISBN 978-1-83769-140-1

For EU product safety concerns:
IN TECH d.o.o., Prolaz Marije Krucifikse Kozulić 3, 51000 Rijeka, Croatia,
info@intechopen.com or visit our website at intechopen.com.

Meet the editor

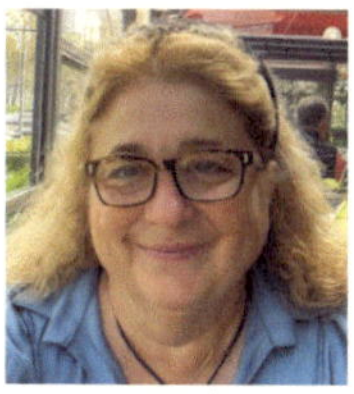

Ayşe Emel Önal, MD, graduated from the Istanbul Medical Faculty, Istanbul University, in 1985. In 1995, she became a public health specialist for the Department of Public Health at the same university. She became an associate professor of public health in 2005 and a full professor in 2011. Currently, she is the director of the Environmental Health Department and the Department of Public Health, Istanbul University. She has more than 300 publications and presentations in national and international journals and congresses to her credit. She has also authored book chapters and served as a book editor. Her main research areas are infectious and chronic non-communicable diseases, epidemiology, gerontology, and environmental health.

Contents

Preface

In primary care, general practitioners and nurses generally protect the health of individuals and treat acute diseases. Doctors who specialize in secondary health care treat patients in secondary-level hospitals. In tertiary care, highly specialized equipment and health professionals provide health care. Tertiary care is specialized care provided in secondary or tertiary-level hospitals or similar specific centers. Tertiary care often requires highly specialized doctors, medical experts, and equipment to care for serious or life-threatening illnesses. These situations may include, for example, congenital malformation, coronary artery bypass surgery, dialysis, serious head injuries, abdominal injuries, undiagnosed clinical conditions, plastic and reconstructive surgeries, brain surgery, serious burn treatments, eye surgeries, and complicated births. The necessary equipment and environmental and psychosocial environment must be provided for these interventions.

This book includes nine chapters organized into five sections.

Section 1: "Definition of Tertiary Health Care"

Chapter 1: "Redefining Tertiary Care in India"

Section 2: "Psychosocial Care in Tertiary Level Hospitals"

Chapter 2: "Psychosocial Care"

Section 3: "Delivery of Treatment Services in Tertiary Care"

Chapter 3: "Delivery of Pharmaceutical Care at Tertiary Level: From Admission to Home Care"

Chapter 4: "Microbial and Parasitic Infections in Tertiary Care: Diagnosis, Treatment, and Prevention Strategies"

Chapter 5: "Diabetic Macular Edema, Clinicopathologic and Keys for Management"

Chapter 6: "Current Perspective on the Treatment of *Helicobacter pylori* Infection"

Section 4" Medical Health Care in Tertiary Level Hospitals"

Chapter 7: "Bowel Preparation before Elective Colorectal Surgery: Its Current Role"

Chapter 8: "Post-Prostatectomy Urinary Incontinence"

Section 5: "Improving the Hospital Environment"

Chapter 9: "The Environmental Impact on Advanced Midwives from Underutilization in Tertiary Hospital"

With its comprehensive examination of tertiary health care and relevant case examples, this book is a useful resource for health professionals. I would like to thank all the chapter authors and the IntechOpen technical team.

Ayşe Emel Önal, M.D.
Professor,
Istanbul Medical Faculty,
Department of Public Health,
Istanbul University,
Istanbul, Türkiye

Section 1

Definition of Tertiary Health Care

Chapter 1

Redefining Tertiary Care in India

Kallakuri Sailaja and P.V. Buddha

Abstract

Tertiary care is the apex of health care pyramid. Usually patients with congenital or unidentified medical conditions present to the tertiary care. Rest are those after an index admission, enter into multiple unpredictable complications. Multidisciplinary approach with 'fresh' thought process is vital. Integrated skills and comprehensive knowledge are important. By the time patient presents to tertiary care patient as well as attendees will be in severe depression with added financial constraints. This contributes to compromise of host immunity. Henceforth a psychosocial support system with empathy is necessary. What went wrong is not always the relevant question, how things can be improved is the pertinent point.

Keywords: redefining tertiary healthcare, self-sustenance, infrastructure planning, referral system, psychosocial aspects of tertiary care

1. Introduction

India is a vast country with varied geographical, cultural and economic zones. Seven and half decades after gaining independence and two years after Covid pandemic, India stands as one of the most viable healthcare delivery systems in the world. Modified universal immunization policy is a major preventive strategy of the Indian public health care system at primary level. Grass root personnel involved have done their best in delivery of Covid vaccination also. The speed and alacrity with which they took digital format of work is highly commendable.

National health policy 2017 has set the vision and tone for achieving universal health coverage. National Health Mission (NHM) adopted a primary health care program with the establishment of Health and Wellness Centers (HWCs)

Now the need of the hour is to redefine the provision of tertiary care to the general population.

2. Present scenario and scope of tertiary care in India

In India the chronic and non-communicable diseases account for 53% of all deaths and 44% of disability adjusted life years [1].

Diabetes, cardiovascular, liver and kidney diseases, autoimmune diseases, blood dyscrasias, muscular and rheumatic ailments are all included in this category [2].

Added to this, is rising incidence of trauma cases due to the rise in daily journeys of the general public by road, rail and air ways.

	Males	Females	Both
Population	3,929,973,836	3,864,824,712	7,794,798,844
New cases	10,065,305	9,227,484	19,292,789
Age standard incidence rate	222.0	186.0	201.0
Risk of developing <75 yrs.%	22.6	18.6	20.4
No. of cancer deaths	5,528,810	4,428,323	9958,133
Age-standardized mortality rate	120.8	84.2	100.7
Risk of dying before 75 yrs.%	12.6%	8.9%	10.7%
5 yr. prevalent cases	24,828,480	25,721,807	50,550,287
Topmost frequent cancers excluding non-melanoma skin cancers	Lung, prostate, colorectum, stomach, liver	Breast, colorectum, lung, cervix uteri, thyroid	Breast, lung, colorectum, prostate, stomach

Table 1.
Summary cancer statistics 2020, world [3].

	Males	Females	Both
Population	717,100,976	662,903,415	1,380,004,378
New cases	646,030	678,383	1,324,413
Age standard incidence rate	95.7	99.3	97.1
Risk of developing <75 yrs.%	10.4	10.5	10.4
No. of cancer deaths	438,297	413,381	851,678
Age-standardized mortality rate	65.4%	61.0%	63.1%
5 yr. prevalent cases	1,208,835	1,511,416	2,720,251
Topmost frequent cancers excluding non-melanoma skin cancers	Lip, oral cavity, lung, stomach, colorectum, esophagus	Breast, cervix utere, ovary, lip, oral cavity, colorectum	Breast, lip, oral cavity, cervix uteri, lung, colorectum

Table 2.
Summary cancer statistics 2020, India [4].

Cancer cases have increased throughout the world due to both increased incidence and early detection combined with awareness among general public. In the year 2020 the global burden of cancer rose to an estimated 19,292 million new cases with 9958 million deaths (**Table 1**) [3].

In India in the year 2020, the number of prevalent cases (5 years) is about 2,720,251, the number of new cases 1,324,413 and the number of deaths 851,678 (**Table 2**) [4].

Each of the above category needs tertiary care and support thus elevating the need for dedicated health care delivery centres.

3. Overview

By definition, 'tertiary care' program has to include complex diagnostic procedures and treatment modalities to be performed by medical specialists in state of the art facilities. All the acute trauma, emergency cases and chronic disabling diseases need tertiary care setup.

The Government of India has taken up in 2021, the norm of establishing one medical college for every district in the country. This has created a great buzz in medical education and health-care delivery across the length and breadth of the country. It will ensure adequate training of medical students as well as availability of specialist services to the general public. But the vital role of infrastructure to diagnose, stage and treat chronic diseases cannot be taken lightly. From the inception level tertiary care needs proper planning, dedicated execution, and feedback based follow up for a successful functioning.

Hitherto in India, Tertiary Care Centers functioned in the form of institutions with autonomous protocol like the Tata Memorial Centre for cancer—Mumbai, Adayar Cancer Centre—Chennai, Aravind Eye Care—Madurai, Christian Medical Centre—Vellore, AIIMS—Delhi, PGI—Chandigarh, Jipmer—Pondicherry, Railway and Defense Hospitals, etc. In the past three decades a chain of private healthcare delivery institutions have come up with international standards in investigative facilities and top notch efficient individuals working round the clock. A syndrome based diagnosis and management have contributed to many miracles in saving the precious lives of millions of patients. Research work regarding disease pattern, innovative design in rehabilitation programs viz. Jaipur foot, low cost laparoscopic instruments, Continuous Medical Education have been pursued by these institutes rising up to international standards. Medical tourism was also a part of this.

To bring these facilities to the public at large is a tough task. With rising cases of organ compromise and failure such as kidney, liver, lung and heart even special procedures like dialysis and organ transplantation surface to the front line.

Further there is a rising incidence of congenital anomalies including autism, pediatric illnesses and cancer cases. Henceforth it is a challenge to channelize the medical personnel as well as infrastructure and make it available for the reach of an average Indian patient.

In this chapter the medical, psychosocial and environmental aspects of tertiary care are discussed along with the pertinent question why tertiary care in India needs to be redefined?

A set of proposals are also recorded herewith as a Model for Modern Tertiary Care Centre Protocol (MTCCP) for future reference and direction.

The most important principle to run a Tertiary Care Centre is to have a proper referral system. This should not be violated by any means and should be strictly adhered to.

Tertiary care means not only specialist care but also disease specific care. Hence a proper referral system will ensure targeted patient care both therapeutic and support care.

3.1 Medical facilities

The medical facilities necessary for tertiary care can be divided under three headings.

A. Infrastructure.

B. Diagnostic facilities.

C. Staff/personnel.

3.1.1 Infrastructure

Accessibility of tertiary care at district headquarters is vital. The designing, construction and maintenance of all the buildings in the facility is the responsibility of the infrastructure development wing of that State. The MTCC shall be maintained as per NABH and NMC guidelines currently in vogue. Budgetary allocations for infrastructure shall be independent of the annual budget for patient care.

Currently, the teaching hospitals affiliated to medical colleges are being regarded as Tertiary Care Centers. In reality they are not. They do not have a uniform plan either in buildings, specialist departments and super specialties departments. A wide variation in the establishment of most vital services has given place to uneven distribution of specialist care resulting in deprivation of essential services to the patients of that region.

For example, in one of the states two medical colleges each of more than five decades of existence, just 150 km away from each other, differ in departments of Cardiology, Gastroenterology, Nephrology in Medical specialty and functioning Cardiothoracic surgery in Surgical specialty even now. This discrepancy jeopardizes the patient care, treatment methods, professional skills and even the academic teaching between the two institutes.

Diseases of one zone are no less in severity than the other zone. Even the student who seeks admission after all the hardships of appearing for a National level Qualifying entrance examination is denied Learning experience grossly for no fault of his/her. The state Government, State and National medical councils along with the elected representatives of that area have no understanding of this major problem. It is always looked upon as the inefficiency and lack of resourcefulness of the concerned medical college staff, Principal and hospital administration that are responsible for this gulf. This is a sad state of affairs.

That's why, it is imperative that a National Level Modern Tertiary Care Centre Protocol (MTCCP) must be contrived and be put into practice by the Government.

redefining tertiary care means.

1. Elimination of disproportionate distribution of medical services.

2. Bringing specialized medical care to the general public.

This needs a thorough scrutiny of available infrastructure, working conditions of the already established specialty services and correction of the gaps. Organization of Tertiary Care Centre can be modified to offer clinical research and training programs. This authenticates the function in a better way.

Usually institutes are burdened with dedicated teaching programs. Teaching includes student evaluation also. Such an academic course in progress, may compromise the attention and energies of the professionals. Indian Government Hospitals do a lot of work but lack in documentation and follow up. Many smaller countries like Japan and Arab countries have contributed to good number of activities such as clinical and treatment protocol trials and research. India lacks in standardization of work. This should be corrected.

Moreover, the existing teaching hospital buildings are terribly congested and do not have enough space for modern arrangement of wards. They are not having technical support to tackle sanitation and electricity needs for intensive care units and laboratories to perform the specific investigations. They also lack in communications and digital networks for e-hospital administration and services. Lack of ventilation, space for attendants, facilities for differently abled personnel are gross defects to be considered.

Every time an Accreditation Team arrives the inspection is done with much compromise with regards to disposition, emergency services and many a time monitoring staff. This type of window dressing cannot be taken to be any progress or up gradation.

The NABH protocol directed Ward Carts, ICU and Operation Theater design and even sterilization measures followed presently are inadequate. So, we propose a dedicated Tertiary Care Center (TCC) to be constructed. The tertiary care system in other countries needs to be viewed at this juncture.

Hospitals and clinics can be broadly categorized by the organizations that manage them.

In the country of Japan the healthcare delivery system is a mixture of both private and governmental organizations. Corporate clinics are gaining more prominence in recent times. This resembles that of the Indian Health care delivery system. The types of hospitals operating in Japan include general hospitals, advanced treatment hospitals, regional support hospitals, clinical research hospitals, psychiatric hospitals and tuberculosis hospitals. Thus, it can be observed that a specific disease based hospital care is being practiced. Among these general hospitals will differ from the rest by the staffing pattern. Those which fulfilled the staffing pattern may be licensed to operate.

In Japan the hospital beds are classified as general psychiatric infectious disease tuberculosis and long term care beds. Thus, there is a disease specific organization of beds. Even in the number of hospital beds there are large disparities for patient's choice. For example, when studied in Kochi prefecture, the number of hospital beds is about three times higher in comparison with Kanagawa prefecture where it is the lowest [5].

The healthcare scenario in China is somewhat similar to that in India. Patients are not forced in their selection of admission in Medical Institutes, so they go to the nearest and cheaper institutes than attend a tertiary hospital. Thus in China the necessity for a tiered healthcare delivery policy to differentiate the function of hospitals is not yet implemented. A tiered healthcare delivery system seems to become a vital element of China's Healthcare reforms in the coming years. An average Chinese citizen is free to select a medical institution of their choice and they have the policy of offering various cover ratios for patients admitted to different levels of hospitals. The highest 'coverage ratio' means the lowest self payment ratio for patients in primary hospitals. The and lowest cover ratio for patients in tertiary hospitals means the highest self payment ratio.

In the majority of hospitals in other countries such as the United Kingdom and France are public facilities [6].

A well drafted research paper with inputs regarding hospital infrastructure was previously proposed by Devanshi Gaur et al. [7] and gives an innovative planning of tertiary care hospital along with the probable challenges there of.

Establishment of TCC:

Infrastructure: Establishment of the hospital at a pre-planned place in the vicinity of city limits will encourage the growth of a satellite township. In such a scenario various consumer services will flourish. This can be converted to a source of income generation and financial self-support. A medical hub ensures multi-specialty medical care to the target population.

An all-inclusive premise for a Tertiary Care Center is a better idea and is not impossible to plan and construct.

A well-conceived plan shall augur a better environment for future challenges in terms of changing patterns of diseases and medical emergencies.

With advancements in technology a TCC will soon emerge as the best service nodal point for the needs of the ever evolving society. Multinational company office buildings and commercial centers like shopping malls and Inox theaters are being erected in a matter of months. So, a properly planned hospital can as well be planned. A positive initiative and execution will definitely make it a reality.

In India 'Arc model' or 'U' shaped accessibility to a series of buildings is rarely followed.

Blind ends, crises-crossing of roads with unlicensed encroachments, unauthorized parking of vehicles is the major constraint even within premises.

Huge congestion of vehicles, drugs and consumables vehicles, and ambulances is a daily occurrence.

One main and common approach road with bylines for each wing of the hospital like emergency, mass casualties, and trauma etc. at the designing stage itself is preferable. Provision for airlift is important for patients brought from far off places and also for organ retrieval and donation which needs green corridor. This has been already provided in some of the state TCCs with the initiative of the local state government.

Buildings of definite standards, electrification and provision for generators or solar power plants are necessary. Recent civil construction methodology has changed by leaps and bounds to evolve into cost-effective and strong structure (**Figure 1**).

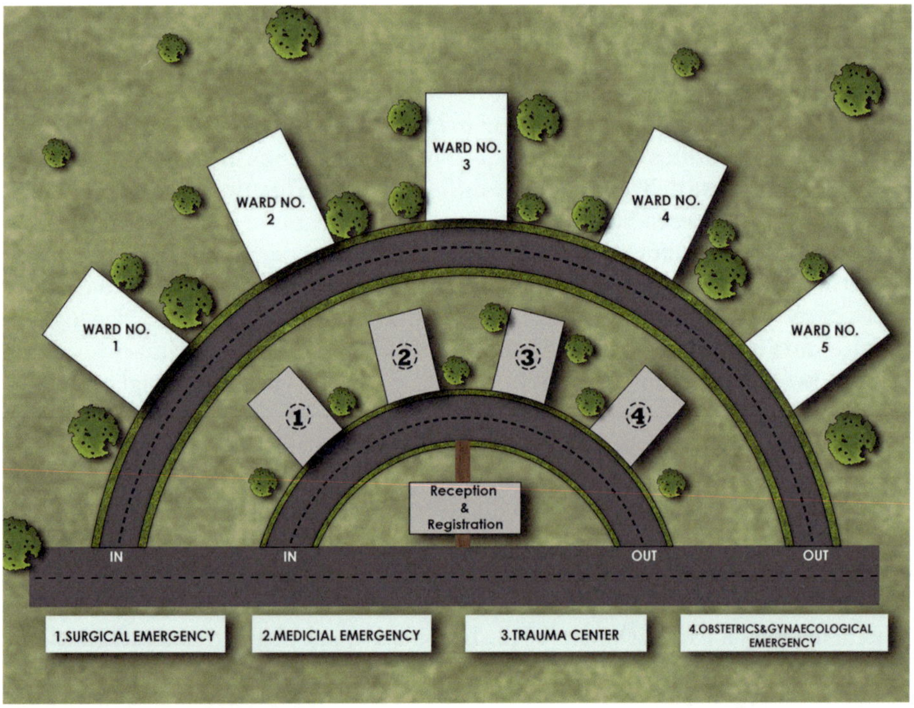

Figure 1.
Proposed model for Hospital Building.

The bureaucratic delays and over shooting of time schedules is on one side while compromise in standards is on the other side to be tackled firmly. Stringent measures regarding quality control is important.

A list of diseases in order of complexity and chronicity that are referred to the TCC is to be prepared to streamline the case load.

The present Ayushman Bharat program identified the organization of healthcare service delivery with chronic illnesses follow up at Health and Wellness Centers (HWCs) on specific days of the week and referral of patients by the medical officer in charge either physically or through telephonic consultation.

This has to be very strictly followed to the tune that both physical and digital deviation is not possible. Then only the target population is eligible to visit Tertiary Care Centers for specific purposes.

Screening at the outset at the reception area will filter the patients to ensure that specialist care services and bed occupancy are not compromised or misutilised. A definite referral shall be the sole eligibility criterion for further evaluation.

Emergency & casualty for trauma with blood bank and radiology services, casualty for other than trauma cases with emergency operation theaters and 24 h laboratory, dedicated wing for MCH.

(Mother and child health care services) building and intensive care units (ICUs) are all to be planned as an arc with interconnecting walkover bridges having wheelchair or trolley friendly facilities.

Patient transport should be in the form of ramps with proper wall support. Solar/battery driven buggy facility is very vital to ease the transport within premises.

The ground floor is ideal for emergencies, trauma, attached laboratory, basic radiology. First, second and third floors can be planned for wards. Elevator facilities like in commercial centers can be provided for staff and patients separately.

All wards need a central nursing station with emergency cart, basic laboratory, mobile X-ray plant and emergency ultrasound machine for utilization.

Resuscitation units must be provided for every section containing bed strength of 50.

Protected water supply and restroom maintenance is to be taken care of. Fire safety outlets and measures to prevent or limit spread of fire are to be installed.

Bedside oxygen supply is to be centralized and be provided with frequent safety checks. The present measures have been installed in a hasty manner during Covid pandemic and they are not being maintained and checked periodically.

Self-sufficiency in power generation and waste disposal is very vital. This self-sustenance can be ushered in by establishment of biogas plant, solar panels, wind energy as part of infrastructure. Sewage disposal, disposal of wound dressings, bed rolls and diapers is to be given paramount importance so as to prevent recycling of infected materials. Safe disposal of sharp needles and body parts has to be scientific.

We propose a Government run biomedical waste disposal unit (BMWD unit) with proper affiliation to pollution control board for every district. This shall replace the present private organizations taking advantage of the monetary benefits yet with disposal norms which are never under proper scrutiny. Bringing all the private health care delivery units under this Government run BMWD unit will have standardization of disposal with revenue generation by channelization of services. Similar to the Motor Vehicle act a BMWD act can be brought into existence and taxation of small clinics to corporate hospital units will pave the way for a healthy country.

Quality control measures with follow up and scrutiny is the need of the hour. Unfortunately, occasional news of hazards regarding disposal of blood stained linen and body parts or dead fetuses is considered sensational. But a practical solution has not been proposed or implemented. Hence a judicious daily clearance shall make a better environment.

The gap between proposals and implementation is often large and remains unbridged over decades. In fact, the proposal to make Tertiary care a public-private partnership and the challenges there of have been discussed in great detail by previous research workers also [7]. Any proposal needs a governmental initiative and strict scrutiny is a must. Institutes need leaders and leaders make institutes, thus finding a right combination is vital.

3.1.2 Database

A central operating system of registration and Health Unique Identity Number is to be developed for database registration. This UID can be developed at the primary health center to be quoted in the referral or it can be provided as personal information at the TCC. Linking Aadhar numbers is the best way to retrieve or enter health information for the individual thus every citizen is allotted a Health Unique ID for his life. Once such a system comes into vogue, Health Insurance can also be streamlined.

The internet facility of the hospital must be ensured by a central operating system with LAN connections and proper backup. Automation in filling up details will ensure data entry and retrieval becomes easy and will be having accountability with regard to services offered. This is not a big issue as such a system is already in vogue for large hotels and tourist places. The same model can be studied to apply in health care.

3.1.3 Diagnostic facilities

Doctor and nursing staff in treating a patient entirely depend upon the investigative procedures and their results. Most of the times daily monitoring and on the spot verification of blood parameters marks the key step to plan and continue treatment schedules. This is the major breakeven point of defining morbidity and mortality of a patient. Multi monitors, autoanalyzers, automatic alarms are all the paraphernalia in decision making for the correct initiation of treatment and changes thereof.

Clinical laboratories presently in Government setup are bereft of basic machinery like auto analysers. Sometimes the outsourcing services supply incompatible reagents and test kits with lacs of rupees being wasted just due to lack of knowledge regarding the machine make and version. Microbiology and Pathology investigations need more sensitive equipment with regard to sterile area and culture sensitivity test resources. This loophole has to be corrected by providing.

1. Ward wise sample collection points.

2. Wing wise technicians to conduct the tests and.

3. Specialty wise reporting authority.

4. And last but not the least a time bound monitoring facility for checking the quality assurance and actual availability of supplements.

Follow up should be on daily stock verification and automatic supply of reagents basing on case turnover. This will correct non-availability of various investigations in the hospital premises which encourages third party encroachments with investigation mafia.

The establishment of above facilities should correlate with the bed strength similar to the doctor-patient, nurse-bed ratios.

The intensive care units for each wing need to be operational round the clock and hence strengthened by both equipment and staff adequately.

Yet another important aspect of diagnostic facilities is the procurement of radiation based investigative machinery. X-ray plants, CT & MRI machinery need to be established separately for medical and surgical patients ensuring less confusion and waiting period. Reporting of these investigations is already being outsourced by tale radiology hence will be totally comfortable for the specialists. The same principle can be followed.

In the present scenario the number of tests done usually does not match the genuine number of investigations ordered by the treating doctors. This leads to off the record exposure leading to criminal wastage of the facility and black marketing of the tests. A callous attitude with regard to siphoning of costly investigations dents the system heavily and is a painful truth to be accepted in Government hospitals. This pilferage of services is to be firmly handled with due penalties to usher in foolproof practices.

Apart from this, interventional radiology procedures are of great importance which save lives and provide minimum access methods with maximum benefit for patients for certain diseases. These are to be treated on par with ICU and emergency care. This point is to be included in the plan of the construction and establishment.

Oftentimes there is a news article about rats in ICUs and failed radiology services. It is the system which fails to function, but not the duty doctor, nurse or technician.

The investigation facilities form the core of the functionality of the TCC which needs to have a separate biotechnology wing for repairs, replacements and maintenance.

Social responsibility of large scale industries in the local area can contribute to the maintenance of this wing.

3.1.4 Staff and personnel

Staff pattern in a Tertiary Care Center will be in three tiers.

3.1.4.1 Non-medical

Maintenance staff are for cleaning and disposal, laundry, staff to deliver drugs, dressings etc., security guards, reception and registration with 'May I Help you' cubicle, pantry and bedside help.

A novel approach is to have a volunteer wing. A possible liaison with the local medical and paramedical students' wings, social service organizations will definitely go a long way to fill the gaps rather than prolonged periods of no or less attention to the needy patients.

Mechanization of cleaning and laundry is to be installed. Establishment of semi-automatic washing machines with driers is quite practicable.

3.1.4.2 Nursing

Ensuring adequate staff is of utmost importance with allowance of leave pattern for a 8 h of daily duty or 50 h per week. A proper central body has to monitor the attendance. Automatic punching systems can streamline the staff capacity.

Proper duty rooms, dress changing facility with provision of food during duty hours can encourage better efficiency. Group drills, six monthly audits will ensure more participation with assurance of workplace dignity.

One kitchen for one specialty wing is the best method to take care of the needs of patients as well as the staff. Apart from this, provision of restaurants for access to the public will encourage revenue generation.

3.1.4.3 Medical specialists

Hitherto all days in a week are taken to be working days for the professionals to look after and follow up out-patients and in-patients. However, this can be modified as weekdays (5) and weekend days (2) to have uniformity in the care. Doctors can be rotated in their weekdays and weekend duties. This will ensure a better orientation and mental readiness to discharge medical officer duties. Accountability and follow up of the cases will be definitely better by this process.

Registered medical doctors with their specialty will encourage a proper direction of the patients to the concerned specialization.

A tier system with teams for each ward will ensure each professional to work with responsibility. A service track record shall be maintained which will keep track of the number of working hours and the quality of work done. This will in a way define each doctor, nursing assistant and technician based on their work output to have bonus or elevation.

The present method of promotion to a higher cadre brings in non-functional senior staff members drawing better salary based on their number of years in service rather than work output. This must be ended.

3.2 Psycho social

The Tertiary Care Centers (TCC) is not mere treatment centers. They are evaluation and rehabilitation centers. The psycho social needs of patients who come here are completely different from those present to regular hospitals.

A terminal illness, an incapacitating neuromuscular disability, mental retardation, organ failure and cancer are some of the examples which need a lot of emotional and moral support.

Inpatients tend to develop intensive care unit psychosis, post trauma psychosis, fear of death and deformity, depression due to prolonged course of the disease, mood swings and anger towards fellow human beings. All these have been described. But, these were given no importance all these years. The appropriate role of psychologist, psychiatrist, nursing assistant, physio therapist, trainer, stoma care specialist and nutritionist has been neglected beyond measure especially in the government set up. This gap is to be filled carefully and with proper and professional planning and by team approach.

Proper suggestions for rehabilitation and reorientation of daily life are to be given to the patients. Post procedural handouts, videos, oral explanation by nursing assistants will make paramount change in the otherwise handicapped life of the physiotherapy plays an important role.

Home care in terms of nursing and medical care of patients with prolonged illnesses is to be integrated to the respective departments. For this training of attendants is vital.

Psychologists, facilitators and self-help groups are important.

The rehab team shall have an overall picture and review of the patient before discharge.

Follow up by video call or visit can be done.

It needs weeks to months or sometimes years to reach a plateau in the sinuous ups and downs in the natural history of prolonged illnesses.

3.3 Environmental

Proper ventilation and air entry is to be ensured. Stringent practices of sanitation and sterilization must be followed. Greenhouse effect by channelizing the sunlight through shades and curtains, increasing indoor plants, ensuring green zones between wards and buildings, rainwater recycling, sewage water disposal are a must.

Plastic ban with usage of native natural materials like leaves and tree bark will help reduce carbon waste. Drainage system is a far cry in the present setup which needs proper planning. Night time ventilation is defective in most of the institutions.

Rainy season is another big challenge in maintenance of sanitation and cleanliness.

Smiling nursing staff who greet the patient is almost unknown in the government sector. This change in the psyche of Indian Government Service is in fact a big lacuna.

Poverty and illiteracy can no longer be the pretext for a proper provision of the above measures. Availability and enforcement is the need of the hour. Health care delivery system is to be given the status of a medium scale Industry with definite budget allocations and scrutiny.

A healthy population will contribute better for the economy growth. Quality assurance is not by too many rules. It has to follow a flow chart of diagram.

Centralized monitoring and correction of loopholes alone will ensure a fresh beginning for health care delivery.

Employee unrest with paucity of regular payment of salaries and monetary benefits is very common over all these years.

A definitive Human Resources Management needs better funds allocation.

Railways, the largest national institution under the central government has witnessed a big leap forward in standards and modern style of functionality. Similarly, a proactive approach is necessary in health care also.

4. Conclusions

A new idea is never a waste. It is built upon previous failures and deficits. Like Metro facilities in Indian Cities, Modern Tertiary Care Centers (MDTCCs) a fresh thought process is necessary. A systematic review paves the way to a better version of planning.

It is always good to correct and proceed hopefully than to be silent and carry on with the old and outdated system.

We sincerely hope to have the establishment of a model and operationally practical Tertiary Care Center.

5. Proposals

1. Tertiary care can be given the status of medium scale industry by Constitutional Amendment.

Health and education form the backbone of the country. They ensure the future of society.

Health care delivery system has intrinsic financial stability by way of medical insurance, promotes a lot of employment opportunities and accommodates the best professionals, hence a viable system.

2. The medical research in India needs to be given a judicious place once TCC is available.

3. Medical tourism wherein either Non-resident Indians or Foreign patients undergo treatment will be a new facet for the Indian economy. It ensures foreign currency flow by giving the advantage of low cost, high precision quality medical care.

We have high hopes regarding radical change in the outlook towards tertiary care in India when dedicated implementation of standards.

Acknowledgements

We thank Mr. A.S.N. Rao for his help in typing work.

Acronyms and abbreviations

NABH	National Accreditation Board for Hospitals and Health Care Providers
ICU	intensive care unit
MTCC	Modern Tertiary Care Centre
TCC	Tertiary Care Centre
HWHC	Health and Wellness Centres
MCH	Maternal and Child Health Care
BMWD unit	biomedical waste disposal unit
UID	Unique Identification Number
LAN	local area network

DOI: http://dx.doi.org/10.5772/intechopen.112750

Author details

Kallakuri Sailaja[1]* and P.V. Buddha[2]

1 DNB General Surgery, Rangaraya Medical College, Kakinada, India

2 Saikrupa Clinic, Kakinada, India

*Address all correspondence to: sailaja7074@gmail.com

References

[1] Global Cancer Observatory, IARC-International Agency for Research on Cancer (Online database). The Global Cancer Observatory. 2020

[2] Gondal V. 5. Health status of India. 5b. Lifestyle diseases. In: Lifestyle Diseases on the Rise in India. IndiaFit Report. 2022-2023. p. 26. Available from: https://db.india.gov.in.chronic diseases lifestyle

[3] World Health Organisation, Global Cancer Observatory. 2020

[4] Globocan. The Global Cancer Observatory. Factsheet, India. 2020

[5] Japan Health Policy Now JHPN-4.2: Medical Facilities and Hospital Beds in Japan. Available from: https://japanhpn.org/en/section4.2

[6] Chu Y, Tao H, Sendi P. Detecting undifferentiation of tertiary and county hospitals in China in adoption of DRG instrument. Healthcare (Basel). 2021;**9**(8):922. DOI: 10.3390/healthcare9080922

[7] Gaur D, Paul VK, Judson L, Basu C. Department of Building Engineering and Management, School of Planning and Architecture, New Delhi, India

Section 2

Psychosocial Care in Tertiary Level Hospitals

Chapter 2

Psychosocial Care

Lucy Matsayi Aji, Ahmad Baba Muhammad and Hassan Abubakar

Abstract

Psychosocial care refers to the provision of emotional, social, and spiritual support to individuals or groups of people who are experiencing psychological or emotional distress, such as anxiety, depression, grief, trauma, or chronic illness. This type of care aims to promote the individual's mental health and well-being by addressing the psychological and social factors that may contribute to their distress and by helping them, develop coping skills and strategies to manage their emotions and behaviors. Psychosocial care can be provided by a variety of healthcare professionals, including psychologists, psychiatrists, social workers, counselors, and nurses, among others. It can take many forms, such as individual or group therapy, cognitive-behavioral therapy, art therapy, mindfulness-based interventions, and support groups. The ultimate goal of psychosocial care is to help individuals regain a sense of control and meaning in their lives, enhance their quality of life, and improve their overall mental health and well-being.

Keywords: psychosocial care, component of psychosocial care, mental health conditions, coping skills and strategies, types of therapies

1. Introduction

Psychosocial care is a multidimensional approach that involves addressing the emotional, social, and spiritual needs of individuals to promote their mental health and well-being. Psychosocial care is a holistic approach to addressing the emotional, social, and spiritual needs of individuals who are experiencing psychological or emotional distress. Individuals who are experiencing psychological or emotional distress may have a variety of needs related to their emotional, social, and spiritual well-being. It is important to recognize that everyone's needs are unique and may change over time. Psychosocial care involves a holistic approach to healthcare that recognizes the interconnectedness of physical, emotional, and social well-being, and seeks to address all aspects of a person's health and well-being. The most effective support will be tailored to the individual and their specific situation [1, 2]. Psychosocial care is based on the notion that mental health is not just the absence of mental illness but also the presence of positive psychological and social well-being. It can help individuals, families, or communities to develop resilience and coping skills to improve their relationships and enhance quality of life.

1.1 Meaning of psychosocial care

Psychosocial refers to "the dynamic relationship between the psychological and social dimension of a person, where one influences the other." The psychological aspects refer to an individual's thoughts, emotions, behaviors, memories, perceptions, understanding, and other mental processes. The social aspects refer to the interaction and relationships among individuals, family, peers, and community [3]. Psychosocial care refers to the provision of support and assistance to individuals who are experiencing mental or emotional distress, or who are dealing with challenging life circumstances. The term encompasses a broad range of interventions that aim to promote mental and emotional well-being, build resilience, and improve the quality of life for those in need. Psychosocial care may involve a variety of approaches, including counseling, psychotherapy, group therapy, support groups, and other forms of emotional and social support. It may be provided by mental health professionals such as psychologists, psychiatrists, and social workers, as well as by trained laypeople and peer support groups. Psychosocial care is often an essential component of the treatment and management of mental health conditions such as depression, anxiety, post-traumatic stress disorder (PTSD), and substance use disorders. However, it can also be valuable for individuals dealing with non-clinical challenges such as grief, relationship issues, and stress related to work or personal life [2].

Psychosocial support: PSS refers to the "processes and actions that promote the holistic wellbeing of people in their psychological and social world. It includes support provided by family and friends" [4]. It can also be described as "a process of facilitating resilience within individuals, families and communities." It is aimed at helping individuals to recover after unpleasant situations or events disrupted their lives and to enhance their ability to return to normality after experiencing adverse events. Psychosocial support as a broad term describes a range of services offered by mental health professionals and other individuals to those in pressing need. Weather designed to help individuals cope with difficult situations, serious illness, or to alleviate distress in whole communities following a disaster, such services may range from mental health counseling, psycho-education, group support to spiritual support and other assistance and are provided by psychologists, social workers, and counselors, among others.

1.2 Examples of needs that may arise

Here are some examples of needs that may arise:

Emotional needs: Individuals in distress may require emotional support to cope with their feelings of anxiety, depression, or other negative emotions. They may need someone to talk to, who can listen without judgment, and offer empathy and validation. They may benefit from therapy or counseling to help them develop coping skills and strategies for managing their emotions [5].

Social needs: Social support is crucial for individuals in distress, as it can help reduce feelings of isolation and loneliness. They may need friends or family members to spend time with, who can offer practical help and emotional support. Support groups can also be beneficial, as they allow individuals to connect with others who are going through similar experiences [6].

Spiritual needs: For some individuals, their spiritual or religious beliefs may provide comfort and meaning during times of distress. They may benefit from speaking with a religious leader or participating in spiritual practices that align with their beliefs. Alternatively, they may find solace in other activities that promote a sense of connection, such as meditation or mindfulness practices [7].

1.3 Component of psychosocial care

Psychosocial care is a type of healthcare that aims to address the emotional, social, and spiritual needs of individuals in addition to their physical needs. It recognizes that a person's mental and emotional well-being is essential to their overall health. According to Nagaswami [8]; Parrish [9]. Here are some components of psychosocial care:

1.3.1 Counseling and therapy

Psychosocial care often involves counseling and therapy to help individuals manage emotional distress and cope with difficult life events. This can include individual therapy, family therapy, group therapy, or support groups. Counseling and therapy are crucial components of psychosocial care. Psychosocial care refers to the support and interventions provided to patients with psychological or social issues that affect their overall well-being. Counseling and therapy involve the use of various techniques and interventions to help individuals improve their mental health and well-being.

Counseling is a process that involves the use of talk therapy to help individuals explore their thoughts, feelings, and behaviors. It is often used to help individuals deal with specific problems, such as stress, anxiety, depression, grief, and relationship issues. Counseling can help individuals develop coping strategies and improve their problem-solving skills, which can help them better manage their emotions and improve their overall mental health.

Therapy, on the other hand, is a more intensive form of counseling that involves working with a trained mental health professional to address more complex mental health issues. Therapists may use a variety of techniques, such as cognitive-behavioral therapy, psychoanalysis, and humanistic therapy, to help individuals address their mental health concerns.

Counseling and therapy are essential components of psychosocial care because they can help individuals improve their mental health and well-being, reduce their symptoms, and improve their quality of life. They can also help individuals develop a better understanding of themselves, their relationships, and their life goals, which can lead to greater personal growth and fulfillment.

1.3.2 Social support

Social support is a crucial component of psychosocial care. It can involve connecting individuals with others who have similar experiences or interests, providing practical assistance, or connecting them with community resources. Social support is a critical component of psychosocial care, as it can have a significant impact on a person's mental health and well-being. Social support refers to the assistance, encouragement, and emotional comfort provided by family, friends, or others in one's social network. Research has shown that individuals who have a strong support system experience better mental health outcomes than those who do not. Social support can provide a sense of belonging, reduce feelings of isolation and loneliness, and increase self-esteem and self-worth. It can also help individuals cope with stressful situations, such as illness or trauma, by providing emotional and practical support.

In the context of psychosocial care, social support can be provided through various interventions, such as support groups, counseling, and peer support programs. These interventions can help individuals build or strengthen their support networks, which can be particularly helpful for those who may not have close family or friends to turn to. It is important for healthcare professionals to recognize the importance of social support and incorporate it into their treatment plans. This may involve connecting patients with support groups or counseling services or working with family and friends to provide ongoing support for the individual. By employing social support as a key component of psychosocial care, healthcare professionals can help improve the mental health and well-being of their patients.

1.3.3 Spiritual care

Spiritual care involves addressing an individual's spiritual needs, whether that involves connecting with a religious or faith community, exploring personal beliefs, or finding meaning and purpose in life.

Spiritual care is another important component of psychosocial care that focuses on the spiritual needs of individuals. It is a holistic approach to care that considers the mind, body, and spirit as interconnected and interdependent parts of a person's overall well-being. Spiritual care can involve a range of practices and interventions, including prayer, meditation, mindfulness, counseling, and pastoral care. It is not limited to any particular religious tradition or belief system, and can be adapted to the individual needs and preferences of each person. Research has shown that spiritual care can have a positive impact on mental health outcomes, such as reducing anxiety, depression, and stress, improving coping skills, and enhancing overall quality of life. Spiritual care can also provide a sense of meaning, purpose, and hope, which can be particularly beneficial for individuals facing serious illnesses, disabilities, or end-of-life care.

In the context of psychosocial care, healthcare professionals can incorporate spiritual care into their treatment plans by working with chaplains, spiritual leaders, or other professionals trained in providing spiritual care. They can also encourage patients to explore their own spiritual beliefs and practices and provide resources and support to help them do so. Spiritual care is an important component of psychosocial care that can help individuals address their spiritual needs and improve their mental health and well-being. By recognizing the importance of spiritual care and incorporating it into their treatment plans, healthcare professionals can provide more holistic and comprehensive care for their patients.

1.3.4 Education and information

Education and information can help individuals understand their illness or condition and make informed decisions about their healthcare. It can also help them develop coping strategies and identify resources and support networks. Education and information can be an essential component of psychosocial care for individuals who are experiencing mental health issues or emotional distress. Providing education and information can help patients better understand their condition, available treatment options, and ways to manage their symptoms.

Education and information can also help to reduce stigma and increase understanding of mental health issues among patients' families and friends. This can help to improve social support and decrease isolation, which can be a significant risk factor for mental health problems. In addition, education and information can empower patients to take an active role in their care, which can lead to better treatment outcomes. This may include providing patients with information about self-care strategies, such as exercise, nutrition, and stress reduction techniques. Education and information are crucial components of psychosocial care that can help patients to better understand their condition, improve their social support, and take an active role in their care, which can lead to better treatment outcomes.

1.3.5 Advocacy

Advocacy involves supporting individuals in navigating the healthcare system, advocating for their rights and needs, and connecting them with resources and services that can help them achieve their goals.

Advocacy can be an important component of psychosocial care for individuals who are experiencing a range of mental health challenges. Psychosocial care is a type of care that addresses both the psychological and social aspects of an individual's life and aims to support their overall well-being. Advocacy refers to the act of supporting and promoting the rights and interests of others. In the context of psychosocial care, advocacy may involve advocating for a patient's right to access appropriate treatment and care, advocating for their right to be treated with dignity and respect, or advocating for their right to make informed decisions about their care.

Advocacy can be provided by mental health professionals, such as therapists or social workers, who work with patients to identify their needs and help them to access appropriate resources and support. Advocacy may also be provided by family members or other support networks who work to ensure that the patient's needs are being met and their rights are being respected. Advocacy can be an important component of psychosocial care, as it can help patients to feel empowered and supported, and can contribute to their overall sense of well-being.

1.3.6 Cultural competence

Cultural competence involves understanding and respecting an individual's cultural background and beliefs, and providing care that is sensitive to their unique needs and experiences.

Cultural competence refers to the ability of healthcare providers to effectively work with individuals from diverse cultural and linguistic backgrounds. As a component of psychosocial care, cultural competence is essential for healthcare providers to understand and respect the cultural beliefs, values, and practices of their patients.

Psychosocial care refers to the psychological and social aspects of healthcare, including emotional support, counseling, and education. It aims to address the emotional and social needs of patients and their families, in addition to their physical health. Cultural competence can enhance the effectiveness of psychosocial care by ensuring that healthcare providers are able to communicate effectively with patients from different cultural backgrounds, understand their unique perspectives and beliefs, and provide care that is respectful and culturally appropriate. It can also help to reduce healthcare disparities, improve patient satisfaction, and promote better health outcomes.

Cultural competence involves ongoing learning and self-reflection, as well as a willingness to adapt to the cultural needs of patients. It requires healthcare providers to recognize and address their own biases and assumptions and to actively seek out opportunities to learn about different cultures and languages. Cultural competence is an important component of psychosocial care, as it can help healthcare providers to provide care that is respectful, effective, and responsive to the needs of their patients from diverse cultural and linguistic backgrounds.

1.3.7 Assessment

The first step in providing psychosocial care is to conduct a comprehensive assessment of the individual's emotional, social, and spiritual needs. This can involve conducting interviews, administering questionnaires, and reviewing medical and psychiatric history. Assessment is a critical component of psychosocial care, as it allows healthcare providers to identify and address the psychological and social needs of patients. Assessment involves gathering information about the patient's mental health, emotional state, social support systems, and any other relevant psychosocial factors that may be affecting their health and well-being.

The assessment process may involve a range of tools and techniques, including clinical interviews, standardized questionnaires, observation, and review of medical records. The healthcare provider may also seek input from family members or other caregivers, as appropriate.

Assessment can help healthcare providers to identify mental health conditions such as depression, anxiety, or post-traumatic stress disorder (PTSD), as well as social factors that may be impacting the patient's health, such as financial stress, social isolation, or lack of access to healthcare resources. This information can then be used to develop a treatment plan that addresses the patient's psychological and social needs.

The assessment also plays an important role in monitoring patient progress over time. By regularly assessing the patient's mental health and social well-being, healthcare providers can determine whether the treatment plan is working and make adjustments as needed. This can help to ensure that patients receive the most effective and appropriate care possible. Overall, assessment is an essential component of psychosocial care, as it allows healthcare providers to understand the unique needs and circumstances of each patient and develop personalized treatment plans that address their psychological and social needs.

1.3.8 Communication

Effective communication is crucial in psychosocial care. Providers should use active listening skills, empathy, and respect to establish a rapport with the individual and facilitate open and honest communication.

Communication is a crucial component of psychosocial care, as it plays a significant role in establishing and maintaining a positive therapeutic relationship between a healthcare provider and a patient. Effective communication can help patients feel heard, understood, and supported, which can lead to improved mental and emotional well-being.

One of the primary goals of psychosocial care is to address the emotional, social, and psychological aspects of a patient's illness or condition. Communication can facilitate this process by providing patients with a safe and supportive environment to express their thoughts and feelings. By actively listening to their patients, healthcare providers can gain a deeper understanding of their needs and concerns, which can help them develop an appropriate care plan that is tailored to the patient's specific needs. Effective communication also involves providing patients with information about their condition, treatment options, and other relevant information that can help them make informed decisions about their care. Healthcare providers can use different communication strategies, such as active listening, empathy, and open-ended questions, to facilitate patient-centered care and encourage patients to participate actively in their treatment.

In summary, communication is a crucial component of psychosocial care as it enables healthcare providers to establish a positive therapeutic relationship with their patients, understand their unique needs and concerns, and provide them with the necessary support and information to make informed decisions about their care.

1.4 Individual or group therapies for mental conditions

According to Churchill et al. [10]; Perry et al. [11]; Thabrew et al. [12]. Both individual and group therapies can be effective in treating mental health conditions, and the choice of which to use may depend on a variety of factors, including the specific condition being treated, the individual's preferences, and the therapist's recommendation.

1.4.1 Individual therapy

It involves working one-on-one with a therapist to address issues related to mental health. This type of therapy can be beneficial for people who prefer to work on their problems in a private setting, or for those who may be uncomfortable sharing their thoughts and feelings in a group setting. Individual therapy can also be tailored to address specific issues that the individual is experiencing, such as trauma, anxiety, or depression.

Individual and group therapies are both valuable approaches for treating mental conditions. Each type of therapy offers unique benefits and is suitable for different situations. Here is an overview of individual and group therapies and their applications:

a. **Psychotherapy/counseling:** This is a one-on-one therapeutic approach where a person works directly with a mental health professional. It allows for a personalized treatment plan tailored to the individual's specific needs.

b. **Cognitive behavioral therapy (CBT)**: CBT focuses on identifying and changing negative thought patterns and behaviors that contribute to mental health issues. It is highly structured and goal-oriented.

c. **Dialectical behavior therapy (DBT):** DBT is often used to treat borderline personality disorder and involves a combination of individual therapy and skills training groups. It emphasizes acceptance and change strategies.

d. **Psychodynamic therapy:** This therapy explores unconscious patterns, past experiences, and the relationship between therapist and client to gain insight into the individual's emotional and psychological well-being.

e. **Eye movement desensitization and reprocessing (EMDR):** Primarily used for trauma-related disorders, EMDR helps individuals process distressing memories and develop adaptive coping mechanisms.

1.4.2 Group therapy

It involves working with a therapist and a group of people who are experiencing similar issues or conditions. This type of therapy can be beneficial for people who may benefit from the support of others who are going through similar experiences. Group therapy can also provide a safe space for individuals to share their thoughts and feelings, receive feedback from others, and develop new coping skills. Ultimately, the decision to pursue individual or group therapy should be based on the individual's unique needs and preferences and should be made in consultation with a qualified mental health professional.

a. **Support groups:** These groups provide a safe environment for individuals facing similar challenges to share experiences, offer support, and learn from one another. Support groups are often led by a facilitator but rely on peer interaction.

b. **Psychoeducational groups:** These groups focus on educating participants about specific mental health conditions or coping strategies. They provide information, teach skills, and encourage discussion and learning.

c. **Process-oriented groups:** These groups allow individuals to explore their thoughts, feelings, and behaviors in a supportive setting. Participants can receive feedback from both the therapist and other group members.

d. **Skills Training groups:** These groups aim to teach specific skills to manage mental health symptoms, such as stress management, social skills, or anger management. The focus is on acquiring practical tools for daily life.

Which approach is most suitable depends on various factors, including the individual's preferences, the nature of their mental condition, and the treatment goals. In some cases, a combination of individual and group therapy may be recommended for comprehensive care. It is important to consult with a mental health professional to determine the best course of treatment for an individual's specific needs.

1.5 Individuals or groups of people who are experiencing psychological or emotional distress

Individuals or groups of people who are experiencing psychological or emotional distress may be going through a range of mental health issues that can affect their well-being and daily functioning. Some common mental health conditions that can cause distress include anxiety disorders, depression, bipolar disorder, post-traumatic stress disorder (PTSD), obsessive-compulsive disorder (OCD), and eating disorders.

It is important to note that everyone experiences mental health differently and that there is no one-size-fits-all solution to addressing mental health concerns. Seeking professional help from a therapist, counselor, or mental health specialist can provide individuals or groups with the support and resources they need to manage their mental health and improve their overall well-being.

1.6 Some common mental health conditions that can cause distress

According to Rosenbaum [13]; Harrison et al. [14]; Trueland [15], there are several common mental health conditions that can cause distress, including:

1. **Anxiety disorders:** Anxiety disorders are characterized by excessive worry, fear, and nervousness that can interfere with daily activities.

2. **Depression:** Depression is a mood disorder that can cause feelings of sadness, hopelessness, and loss of interest in activities.

3. **Bipolar disorder:** Bipolar disorder is a mood disorder characterized by episodes of mania (elevated mood and energy) and depression.

4. **Post-traumatic stress disorder (PTSD):** PTSD is a mental health condition that can develop after a person experiences or witnesses a traumatic event.

5. **Obsessive-compulsive disorder (OCD)**: OCD is a mental health condition that is characterized by obsessive thoughts and compulsive behaviors.

6. **Schizophrenia:** Schizophrenia is a chronic and severe mental disorder that affects how a person thinks, feels, and behaves.

7. **Eating disorders:** Eating disorders are mental health conditions that involve disordered eating behaviors, such as binge eating or purging.

8. **Attention-deficit/hyperactivity disorder (ADHD)**: ADHD is a neuro-developmental disorder that can cause difficulties with attention, hyperactivity, and impulsivity.

These conditions can significantly impact a person's daily life and may require treatment from a mental health professional. There are many different types of mental health conditions that can cause distress, and the signs, symptoms, preventions, and treatments can vary depending on the specific condition. However, here is some general information that may be helpful:

1.6.1 Anxiety disorders

Anxiety disorders are characterized by persistent feelings of fear, worry, or unease. Common types of anxiety disorders include generalized anxiety disorder, panic disorder, social anxiety disorder, and specific phobias. Signs and symptoms may include excessive worry, panic attacks, avoidance of certain situations or activities, and physical symptoms such as sweating, shaking, or rapid heartbeat.

Preventative measures may include stress management techniques such as exercise, relaxation techniques, and healthy lifestyle habits such as proper nutrition and sleep. Treatment options may include therapy, medications, or a combination of both. Anxiety disorders are a group of mental health conditions characterized by persistent feelings of fear, worry, or unease. Common types of anxiety disorders include generalized anxiety disorder, panic disorder, social anxiety disorder, and specific phobias.

Here is some information on the signs, symptoms, preventions, and treatments for anxiety disorders:

1.6.1.1 Signs and symptoms

i. Excessive worry or fear about everyday situations or objects

ii. Panic attacks (sudden and intense feelings of fear or terror)

iii. Avoidance of certain situations or objects

iv. Difficulty concentrating or focusing on tasks

v. Muscle tension or physical symptoms such as sweating, trembling, or rapid heartbeat

vi. Irritability or restlessness

1.6.1.2 Preventative measures

i. Practice stress management techniques such as mindfulness, meditation, or deep breathing exercises

ii. Maintain a healthy lifestyle with regular exercise, a balanced diet, and adequate sleep

iii. Limit or avoid caffeine and alcohol, which can exacerbate symptoms

iv. Avoid or limit exposure to stressful situations or triggers when possible

1.6.1.3 Treatment options

a. **Therapy:** Cognitive-behavioral therapy (CBT) is a common form of therapy used to treat anxiety disorders. CBT helps individuals identify and change negative thought patterns and behaviors that contribute to anxiety symptoms.

b. **Medications:** Antidepressants, such as selective serotonin reuptake inhibitors (SSRIs), are commonly used to treat anxiety disorders. Other medications, such as benzodiazepines, may be prescribed for short-term relief of symptoms.

c. **Self-help strategies:** In addition to seeking professional help, individuals with anxiety disorders may benefit from self-help strategies such as exercise, relaxation techniques, and support from friends and family.

It is important to note that treatment for anxiety disorders can be highly individualized and may involve a combination of different approaches. Seeking professional help from a mental health provider is the best way to determine an appropriate treatment plan.

DOI: http://dx.doi.org/10.5772/intechopen.112016

1.6.2 Depression

Depression is a common mental health condition characterized by persistent feelings of sadness, hopelessness, and lack of interest or pleasure in activities that were once enjoyable. Signs and symptoms may include persistent sadness, feelings of worthlessness or guilt, fatigue, changes in appetite or sleep, and difficulty concentrating.

Depression is a mental health disorder characterized by persistent sadness, loss of interest in activities, changes in appetite, sleep disturbances, fatigue, feelings of guilt or worthlessness, difficulty concentrating, and thoughts of death or suicide. Here are some signs, symptoms, preventions, and treatments for depression:

1.6.2.1 Signs and symptoms

i. Persistent sadness, anxiousness, or feelings of emptiness

ii. Loss of interest or pleasure in activities that were once enjoyed

iii. Difficulty sleeping or oversleeping

iv. Fatigue or decreased energy

v. Changes in appetite and weight

vi. Difficulty concentrating, making decisions, or remembering

vii. Feelings of hopelessness, guilt, or worthlessness

viii. Recurrent thoughts of death, suicide, or suicide attempts

ix. Physical symptoms, such as headaches or digestive problems, that do not respond to treatment

1.6.2.2 Preventions

i. Regular exercise

ii. Healthy diet

iii. Adequate sleep

iv. Limiting alcohol and drug use

v. Managing stress

vi. Staying connected with family and friends

vii. Seeking professional help if needed

1.6.2.3 Treatments

a. **Therapy:** Talking with a mental health professional can help to identify and address the underlying causes of depression, and learn coping skills to manage symptoms.

b. **Medication:** Antidepressant medications, such as selective serotonin reuptake inhibitors (SSRIs), can help to regulate the brain chemicals that affect mood.

c. **Self-care:** Engage in activities that bring pleasure or relaxation, such as exercise, yoga, meditation, or hobbies.

d. **Support groups:** Connecting with others who have experienced depression can provide emotional support and help to reduce feelings of isolation.

It is important to seek help from a mental health professional if you are experiencing symptoms of depression. With proper treatment, people with depression can recover and lead healthy, fulfilling lives.

1.6.3 Bipolar disorder

Bipolar disorder is a mood disorder characterized by periods of intense highs (mania) and lows (depression). Signs and symptoms of mania may include high energy, decreased need for sleep, increased irritability or impulsivity, and grandiose thoughts or delusions. Signs and symptoms of depression may include feelings of sadness, hopelessness, and worthlessness. Preventative measures may include seeking treatment as soon as possible if experiencing symptoms, managing stress, and maintaining a healthy lifestyle. Treatment options may include therapy, medications, or a combination of both. Bipolar disorder is a mental health condition that is characterized by extreme mood swings, ranging from episodes of elevated or manic mood to episodes of depressive mood. Here are some signs, symptoms, preventions, and treatments for bipolar disorder:

1.6.3.1 Signs and symptoms: for bipolar disorder:

i. Manic or hypomanic episode

ii. Elevated, expansive, or irritable mood

iii. Decreased need for sleep

iv. Increased talkativeness

v. Racing thoughts

vi. Distractibility

vii. Increased activity level

viii. Risky behavior

ix. Depressive episode:

x. Depressed mood

xi. Loss of interest or pleasure in activities

xii. Feelings of worthlessness or guilt

xiii. Fatigue or loss of energy

xiv. Insomnia or hypersomnia

xv. Appetite or weight changes

xvi. Thoughts of death or suicide

1.6.3.2 Preventions

Develop a healthy lifestyle: get enough sleep, eat a balanced diet, and exercise regularly.

Avoid drugs and alcohol: they can worsen symptoms and interact with medications.

Keep track of symptoms: it can help identify triggers and patterns.

1.6.3.3 Treatments

Medications: mood stabilizers, antipsychotics, and antidepressants.

Psychotherapy: cognitive-behavioral therapy, family-focused therapy, and interpersonal and social rhythm therapy.

Electroconvulsive therapy (ECT): in severe cases when other treatments do not work.

It is important to seek help if you or someone you know is experiencing symptoms of bipolar disorder. With proper treatment and support, people with bipolar disorder can manage their symptoms and lead fulfilling lives.

1.6.3.4 Obsessive-compulsive disorder (OCD)

OCD is a disorder characterized by recurrent, unwanted thoughts or obsessions and repetitive behaviors or compulsions that are performed in an attempt to relieve anxiety or distress. Signs and symptoms may include repetitive thoughts or behaviors, excessive hand washing, checking behaviors, or organizing and arranging items in a specific way. Preventative measures may include recognizing the signs and symptoms early on and seeking professional help. Treatment options may include therapy, medications, or a combination of both. Obsessive-compulsive disorder (OCD) is a mental health disorder characterized by persistent and intrusive thoughts (obsessions) and repetitive behaviors (compulsions) that individuals feel driven to perform. These obsessions and compulsions can cause significant distress and interfere with daily life.

1.6.3.5 Signs and symptoms of OCD

i. Obsessive thoughts about germs, contamination, or harm to self or others

ii. A need for symmetry or orderliness in everyday life

iii. Compulsive behaviors such as repeated hand-washing, checking and rechecking things, or counting

iv. A sense of anxiety or distress when compulsions are not performed

v. Time-consuming rituals that interfere with daily life, such as spending hours cleaning or organizing

1.6.3.6 Preventive measures for OCD

There is no surefire way to prevent OCD, but early intervention and treatment can help manage symptoms and prevent the condition from becoming more severe.

Stress management techniques such as meditation, yoga, or deep breathing exercises may also help reduce anxiety levels and prevent obsessive thoughts from taking hold.

1.6.3.7 Treatments for OCD

Therapy: Cognitive-behavioral therapy (CBT) is the most effective treatment for OCD. It involves identifying and changing unhealthy thought patterns and behaviors that contribute to OCD symptoms. Exposure and response prevention (ERP) is a specific form of CBT that involves gradually exposing patients to their obsessions and teaching them to resist the urge to perform compulsive behaviors.

Medications: Certain antidepressants, particularly selective serotonin reuptake inhibitors (SSRIs), have been shown to be effective in treating OCD. Other medications, such as antipsychotics, may be used in conjunction with SSRIs for more severe cases.

Deep brain stimulation (DBS): For severe cases, a neurosurgical procedure called deep brain stimulation (DBS) may be an option. This involves implanting electrodes in the brain that stimulate specific areas involved in OCD.

It is important to note that OCD is a chronic condition that requires ongoing management and treatment. People with OCD can benefit from a combination of therapy, medication, and lifestyle changes to help manage their symptoms and improve their quality of life.

1.6.4 Schizophrenia

Schizophrenia is a severe mental illness characterized by disordered thinking, emotions, and behaviors. Signs and symptoms may include delusions, hallucinations, disorganized speech or behavior, and reduced emotional expression. Preventative measures may include seeking treatment as soon as possible if experiencing symptoms and avoiding substance abuse. Treatment options may include therapy, medications, or a combination of both. Schizophrenia is a serious mental illness that affects how a person thinks, feels, and behaves. It is a chronic condition that typically begins in the late teenage years or early adulthood, and it can have a profound impact on a person's ability to function in daily life.

It's important to recognize that mental health conditions can vary widely in their signs and symptoms, and that treatment may involve a combination of different approaches. Seeking professional help as soon as possible can help to manage symptoms and prevent further distress.

1.6.4.1 Here are some signs and symptoms of schizophrenia

1. **Delusions:** False beliefs that are not based in reality, such as thinking that someone is trying to harm you or that you have special powers.

2. **Hallucinations:** Seeing, hearing, or feeling things that are not real, such as hearing voices or seeing people that are not there.

3. **Disordered thinking:** Difficulty organizing thoughts or making logical connections between ideas.

4. **Social withdrawal:** A tendency to isolate oneself and avoid social situations.

5. **Lack of motivation:** A decrease in the ability to initiate and sustain activities or to experience pleasure.

6. **Emotional blunting:** A decrease in the range and intensity of emotions expressed.

1.6.4.2 Some ways to prevent schizophrenia or reduce the risk of developing it include

Avoiding or managing stress: Chronic stress can be a risk factor for schizophrenia, so managing stress through healthy coping mechanisms such as exercise, meditation, or therapy can be helpful.

Avoiding substance abuse: Substance abuse, especially during adolescence, can increase the risk of developing schizophrenia.

Early detection and treatment: Identifying and treating the symptoms of schizophrenia as early as possible can lead to better outcomes and reduce the severity of symptoms.

1.6.4.3 Treatment for schizophrenia

Treatment for schizophrenia typically involves a combination of medication, therapy, and support services. Medications such as antipsychotics can help reduce symptoms such as hallucinations and delusions. Therapy can include cognitive-behavioral therapy or family therapy, which can help patients develop coping skills and improve communication with loved ones. Support services such as case management, vocational training, and housing assistance can help individuals with schizophrenia live independently and improve their quality of life.

It is important to note that schizophrenia is a complex disorder, and treatment may need to be adjusted over time as symptoms and needs change. If you or someone you know is experiencing symptoms of schizophrenia, it is important to seek help from a mental health professional.

1.7 Coping skills and strategies for mental conditions

Coping skills and strategies can be helpful for individuals with mental health conditions to manage their symptoms and improve their overall well-being. It is important to note that coping skills and strategies may vary from person to person and may require trial and error to find what works best for each individual. It is also important to seek professional help if needed and to work with a mental health professional to develop an individualized treatment plan. According to Mindt and Spaulding [16]; Dziegielewski [17]; Silverman [18], here are some coping skills and strategies that may be helpful:

Mindfulness meditation: Mindfulness meditation can help individuals reduce stress, anxiety, and depression symptoms. It involves focusing on the present moment and accepting one's thoughts and feelings without judgment.

Cognitive behavioral therapy (CBT): CBT is a type of therapy that can help individuals identify and change negative thought patterns and behaviors that contribute to mental health conditions.

Exercise: Regular exercise can help improve mood and reduce symptoms of anxiety and depression.

Social Support: Talking with friends, family members, or a mental health professional can provide emotional support and help individuals cope with stress.

Self-care: Taking care of oneself by getting enough sleep, eating a balanced diet, and engaging in activities that bring joy can help improve overall well-being.

Relaxation Techniques: Techniques such as deep breathing, progressive muscle relaxation, and guided imagery can help reduce stress and anxiety.

Art Therapy: Art therapy can help individuals express emotions and process difficult experiences through creative expression.

Medication: For some individuals, medication prescribed by a mental health professional can be an effective way to manage symptoms of mental health conditions.

1.8 Individual or group therapies for mental conditions

Both individual and group therapies can be effective in treating mental health conditions, and the choice of which to use may depend on a variety of factors, including the specific condition being treated, the individual's preferences, and the therapist's recommendation.

Individual therapy involves working one-on-one with a therapist to address issues related to mental health. This type of therapy can be beneficial for people who prefer to work on their problems in a private setting, or for those who may be uncomfortable sharing their thoughts and feelings in a group setting. Individual therapy can also be tailored to address specific issues that the individual is experiencing, such as trauma, anxiety, or depression.

Group therapy involves working with a therapist and a group of people who are experiencing similar issues or conditions. This type of therapy can be beneficial for people who may benefit from the support of others who are going through similar experiences. Group therapy can also provide a safe space for individuals to share their thoughts and feelings, receive feedback from others, and develop new coping skills.

Ultimately, the decision to pursue individual or group therapy should be based on the individual's unique needs and preferences and should be made in consultation with a qualified mental health professional.

2. Types of individual or group therapies for mental conditions

There are several types of individual and group therapies that are commonly used to treat mental health conditions. Here are some of the most common ones:

2.1 Cognitive-behavioral therapy (CBT)

This is a type of talk therapy that focuses on identifying and changing negative thought patterns and behaviors that contribute to mental health problems.

2.1.1 Cognitive-behavioral therapy (CBT) techniques for mental issues

Cognitive-behavioral therapy (CBT) is a type of psychotherapy that has been shown to be effective in treating a variety of mental health issues. It focuses on changing negative thought patterns and behaviors that contribute to these issues. Here are some common CBT techniques:

i. **Cognitive restructuring:** This technique involves identifying and challenging negative thoughts and beliefs that contribute to anxiety, depression, or other mental health problems. The goal is to replace negative thoughts with more positive, realistic ones.

ii. **Behavioral activation:** This technique involves increasing engagement in pleasurable activities and behaviors to improve mood and reduce symptoms of depression.

iii. **Exposure therapy:** This technique involves gradually exposing individuals to situations or stimuli that trigger anxiety or fear in a controlled and safe environment. The goal is to desensitize the individual to these triggers and reduce anxiety.

iv. **Relaxation training:** This technique involves teaching individuals relaxation techniques, such as deep breathing, progressive muscle relaxation, and mindfulness, to reduce symptoms of anxiety and stress.

v. **Problem-solving skills training:** This technique involves teaching individuals how to identify and solve problems that contribute to their mental health issues.

vi. **Social skills training:** This technique involves teaching individuals how to improve their social skills and communication to reduce social anxiety and improve relationships.

These are just a few of the many CBT techniques that can be used to treat mental health issues. The specific techniques used may vary depending on the individual's needs and the type of mental health issue being treated.

2.2 Psychodynamic therapy

This type of therapy focuses on exploring unconscious thoughts and emotions that may be contributing to mental health problems.

2.2.1 Psychodynamic therapy and techniques for mental issues

Psychodynamic therapy is a type of talk therapy that focuses on exploring the unconscious thoughts and emotions that may be contributing to a person's mental health issues. It aims to help individuals gain insight into their thoughts, feelings, and behavior patterns to develop a deeper understanding of themselves and their experiences. Here are some common psychodynamic therapy techniques:

i. **Free association:** This technique involves encouraging individuals to speak freely and spontaneously about their thoughts and feelings without censoring themselves. It can help uncover unconscious thoughts and emotions that may be contributing to mental health issues.

ii. **Dream analysis:** This technique involves exploring the symbols and imagery in an individual's dreams to uncover unconscious thoughts and emotions that may be contributing to their mental health issues.

iii. **Transference:** This technique involves exploring how individuals project their thoughts and feelings onto their therapist, which can provide insights into their relationships and behavior patterns outside of therapy.

iv. **Interpretation:** This technique involves the therapist offering insights and interpretations of the individual's thoughts, feelings, and behavior patterns to help them gain a deeper understanding of themselves.

v. **Working through**: This technique involves helping individuals process and resolve past traumas and emotional conflicts that may be contributing to their mental health issues.

vi. **Therapeutic relationship:** This technique involves developing a strong and trusting relationship between the individual and therapist, which can provide a safe and supportive environment for exploring difficult emotions and experiences.

These are just a few of the many psychodynamic therapy techniques that can be used to treat mental health issues. The specific techniques used may vary depending on the individual's needs and the type of mental health issue being treated.

2.3 Interpersonal therapy (IPT)

This is a type of talk therapy that focuses on improving interpersonal relationships and communication skills. IPT is a structured and evidence-based approach to addressing mental health issues that focuses on improving interpersonal relationships. It can be helpful for a range of mental health conditions, including depression, anxiety, and eating disorders.

2.3.1 Interpersonal therapy (IPT) and techniques for mental issues

Interpersonal therapy (IPT) is a form of psychotherapy that focuses on improving interpersonal relationships and addressing interpersonal problems. It is a time-limited therapy that typically lasts for 12–16 sessions, and it is based on the premise that interpersonal difficulties can lead to mental health issues such as depression and anxiety.

Here are some of the techniques commonly used in IPT to address mental health issues:

a. **Identifying interpersonal issues:** In the initial sessions of IPT, the therapist helps the client to identify the interpersonal issues that are contributing to their mental health issues. This may involve exploring their relationships with family members, friends, romantic partners, and colleagues.

b. **Communication skills training:** IPT may involve teaching clients effective communication skills, such as assertiveness and active listening. These skills can help clients to express their needs and feelings more effectively and improve their relationships.

c. **Role-playing:** In IPT, clients may be asked to role-play interpersonal situations that are causing them distress. This can help them to identify unhelpful patterns of behavior and practice more effective ways of interacting with others.

d. **Problem-solving**: IPT may involve helping clients to identify and solve interpersonal problems. This may include brainstorming solutions to a problem and evaluating the pros and cons of each option.

e. **Grief work:** If a client has experienced a significant loss, such as the death of a loved one or the end of a relationship, IPT may involve helping them to process their grief and adjust to life without the person who has been lost.

2.4 Dialectical behavior therapy (DBT)

This type of therapy focuses on helping individuals regulate emotions and improve relationships by teaching mindfulness, distress tolerance, and interpersonal effectiveness.

2.4.1 Dialectical behavior therapy (DBT) and techniques for mental issues

Dialectical Behavior Therapy (DBT) is a type of therapy that was developed by psychologist Marsha M. Linehan to help people who struggle with emotional dysregulation and difficulty in managing their relationships with others. DBT combines cognitive-behavioral techniques with mindfulness practices to help individuals build skills for emotional regulation, distress tolerance, interpersonal effectiveness, and mindfulness.

Some of the techniques commonly used in DBT include:

a. **Mindfulness meditation:** This technique involves paying attention to the present moment without judgment. Practicing mindfulness can help individuals become more aware of their thoughts and feelings, and learn to regulate them more effectively.

b. **Dialectical thinking:** This technique involves balancing two seemingly opposing ideas or beliefs. By learning to hold both sides of a dilemma or problem, individuals can develop a more balanced and nuanced perspective.

c. **Emotion regulation:** This technique involves learning to identify and manage intense emotions. Techniques for emotion regulation can include mindfulness, distraction, and cognitive restructuring.

d. **Interpersonal effectiveness:** This technique involves learning how to communicate effectively with others, set boundaries, and navigate conflicts.

e. **Distress tolerance:** This technique involves learning to tolerate intense emotions without engaging in harmful behaviors. Techniques for distress tolerance can include distraction, self-soothing, and radical acceptance.

DBT has been found to be effective in treating a range of mental health issues, including borderline personality disorder, depression, anxiety, substance abuse, and eating disorders. It is often used in individual therapy, but can also be delivered in a group setting.

2.5 Family therapy

This type of therapy involves family members in the treatment process to address issues that may be contributing to mental health problems. Family therapy is a type of therapy that involves working with families and couples to improve communication, resolve conflicts, and address mental health issues. The goal of family therapy is to help families develop healthier, more functional relationships and to improve the overall well-being of all family members. Family therapy can be an effective way to address mental health issues and improve family relationships. By working together with a skilled therapist, families can develop new ways of communicating and interacting that can help them to overcome challenges and build stronger, healthier relationships.

2.5.1 Family therapy and techniques for mental issues:

There are many different techniques that can be used in family therapy, depending on the specific needs and goals of the family. Here are a few examples:

i. **Structural family therapy:** This technique focuses on identifying and changing dysfunctional family patterns by reorganizing family roles and boundaries. The therapist may observe family interactions and provide guidance on how to make changes that will improve the family dynamic.

ii. **Strategic family therapy:** This technique involves setting specific goals and developing a plan to achieve those goals. The therapist may assign tasks or give homework to family members to encourage them to make positive changes in their relationships.

iii. **Narrative therapy**: This technique involves exploring the stories and beliefs that families hold about themselves and their relationships. The therapist helps the family to reframe negative stories into more positive and empowering narratives.

iv. **Emotionally focused therapy:** This technique focuses on identifying and addressing emotional barriers that may be preventing family members from connecting with each other. The therapist helps family members to identify and express their emotions in a safe and supportive environment.

v. **Solution-focused therapy:** This technique involves focusing on the solutions rather than the problems. The therapist helps the family to identify what is working well in their relationships and build on those strengths to create a more positive future.

2.6 Group therapy

This type of therapy involves a therapist leading a group of individuals with similar mental health concerns, allowing participants to share experiences and provide support to one another. Group therapy is a type of therapy that involves a therapist leading a group of individuals who share similar mental health issues or concerns. Group therapy provides a safe and supportive environment where individuals can share their experiences, provide feedback, and learn coping strategies from one another.

2.6.1 Group therapy and techniques for mental issues

There are many different techniques used in group therapy, depending on the specific needs and goals of the group. Here are a few examples:

i. **Cognitive behavioral therapy (CBT):** This technique is a goal-oriented therapy that focuses on identifying and changing negative thought patterns and behaviors. The therapist helps group members to recognize unhelpful thoughts and replace them with more positive and adaptive ones.

ii. **Mindfulness-based stress reduction (MBSR):** This technique involves practicing mindfulness meditation and other techniques to reduce stress and promote relaxation. The therapist teaches group members how to focus their attention on the present moment and accept their thoughts and feelings without judgment.

iii. **Interpersonal therapy (IPT):** This technique focuses on improving relationships with others. The therapist helps group members to identify and address relationship problems and learn effective communication skills.

iv. **Dialectical behavioral therapy (DBT):** This technique combines cognitive-behavioral therapy with mindfulness-based techniques to help individuals regulate their emotions and improve their interpersonal skills. The therapist helps group members to identify and change negative thought patterns and behaviors, while also teaching them how to manage their emotions and communicate effectively with others.

v. **Acceptance and commitment therapy (ACT):** This technique focuses on helping individuals develop psychological flexibility by accepting difficult thoughts and emotions and taking action toward their values. The therapist helps group members to identify their values and create goals that align with those values.

Group therapy can be an effective way to address mental health issues and learn coping strategies in a supportive and non-judgmental environment. By working together with a skilled therapist and other group members, individuals can develop new skills and perspectives that can help them to overcome challenges and improve their mental health.

2.7 Art therapy

This type of therapy involves the use of art to help individuals express emotions and improve their mental health. Art therapy is a form of psychotherapy that uses the creative process of art-making to help individuals express and explore their emotions, thoughts, and experiences. It can be a helpful therapeutic intervention for individuals who are experiencing mental health issues, including anxiety, depression, trauma, and stress.

2.7.1 Some techniques commonly used in art therapy include

i. **Drawing or painting**: This can involve using different mediums such as pencils, pastels, watercolors, and acrylic paints to create art that expresses one's emotions and feelings.

ii. **Collage**: This involves combining various materials such as pictures, magazines, and textiles to create a visual representation of one's emotions and experiences.

iii. **Sculpting:** This technique involves molding or shaping clay, play-dough, or other materials to create a three-dimensional representation of one's experiences

iv. **Music therapy:** This involves using music and sounds to help individuals express their emotions and promote relaxation and stress reduction.

v. **Dance therapy:** This involves using movement and dance to help individuals express their emotions, improve their physical and emotional well-being, and promote self-awareness.

Art therapy can be conducted in individual or group settings, and it can be beneficial for individuals of all ages. The goal of art therapy is to help individuals gain insight into their emotions, promote self-expression, and improve their overall mental health and well-being.

2.8 Music therapy

This type of therapy involves the use of music to help individuals express emotions and improve their mental health. Music therapy is a form of therapy that uses music to address the emotional, cognitive, physical, and social needs of individuals. It is an evidence-based practice that can be used to treat a wide range of mental health issues, including anxiety, depression, trauma, and stress.

2.8.1 Some techniques commonly used in music therapy include:

i. **Active music-making:** This involves engaging in activities such as singing, playing instruments, and composing music to express one's emotions and experiences.

ii. **Guided listening:** This involves listening to music that is chosen specifically to evoke certain emotions or feelings, and reflecting on those emotions with a therapist.

iii. **Improvisation:** This involves creating music spontaneously, without pre-planning or rehearsal, as a way of expressing emotions and promoting self-awareness.

iv. **Songwriting:** This involves creating original songs that express one's thoughts, feelings, and experiences.

v. **Movement to music:** This involves using music to facilitate movement and physical expression, which can promote relaxation, stress reduction, and improved emotional well-being.

Music therapy can be conducted in individual or group settings, and it can be beneficial for individuals of all ages. The goal of music therapy is to help individuals gain insight into their emotions, promote self-expression, and improve their overall mental health and well-being. It is important to note that the effectiveness of these therapies may vary depending on the individual and the specific mental health condition being treated. It is best to consult with a mental health professional to determine the most appropriate therapy for a particular situation [12, 18].

3. Conclusions

Psychosocial care plays a vital role in promoting the overall well-being and mental health of individuals. It encompasses a range of interventions and support services aimed at addressing the psychological and social aspects of a person's life. Based on the available knowledge up until September 2021, it is evident that psychosocial care is crucial in various contexts, including healthcare, disaster response, and humanitarian aid. Here are some key conclusions on psychosocial care:

1. **Holistic approach:** Psychosocial care takes a holistic approach to an individual's well-being, considering not only their mental health but also their social,

emotional, and spiritual needs. It recognizes the interconnectedness of these factors and aims to provide comprehensive support.

2. **Mental health promotion**: Psychosocial care plays a significant role in promoting mental health and preventing the development or worsening of mental health disorders. It emphasizes the importance of early intervention, resilience-building, and the development of coping strategies.

3. **Trauma and crisis response:** Psychosocial care is essential in addressing the psychological and emotional needs of individuals who have experienced trauma or crises. It helps individuals process their experiences, manage distressing emotions, and rebuild their lives.

4. **Social support:** Psychosocial care recognizes the importance of social support networks in promoting well-being. It involves fostering social connections, building healthy relationships, and providing opportunities for community engagement, which can enhance resilience and improve mental health outcomes.

5. **Cultural sensitivity:** Effective psychosocial care takes into account cultural, social, and contextual factors. It acknowledges the influence of cultural beliefs, norms, and values on individuals' mental health and tailors interventions accordingly, ensuring cultural sensitivity and respect.

6. **Collaborative approach:** Psychosocial care involves collaboration among various professionals, including psychologists, social workers, counselors, and healthcare providers. It emphasizes interdisciplinary teamwork to provide comprehensive care and support to individuals.

7. **Long-term care:** Psychosocial care recognizes that mental health and psychosocial needs may require ongoing support. It promotes continuity of care and ensures that individuals have access to follow-up services and resources even after the initial intervention.

8. **Prevention and early intervention:** Psychosocial care emphasizes prevention and early intervention strategies to address mental health concerns before they escalate. By promoting mental health literacy, resilience-building, and early identification of risk factors, it aims to reduce the burden of mental health disorders.

In conclusion, psychosocial care is an integral part of promoting mental health and well-being. Its holistic approach, focus on prevention and early intervention, and recognition of social support networks contribute to better mental health outcomes for individuals. Continual research and practice advancements are essential to further improve psychosocial care approaches and ensure that individuals receive the support they need.

Acknowledgements

In order to complete this goal, many people have motivated us. However, we must state that we are exclusively liable for any errors, whether they were caused by omission or commission.

We especially want to thank God Almighty for always being there for us in all facets of life. We owe a debt of gratitude to the administration of Taraba State University and Dr. Adamu N. N., our department head, department of guidance and counseling, Taraba State University, who never gave up trying to lead us cautiously and sagely during the course of doing this study. Their belief in our capacity to carry out a good deed gave us a unique courage to work tirelessly and unabatedly on this book. Despite having busy schedules, they were always there to help us. This work has been made possible by their dedication, cordial criticism, cooperation, and moral support.

Conflict of interest

"The authors declare no conflict of interest".

Author details

Lucy Matsayi Aji*, Ahmad Baba Muhammad and Hassan Abubakar
Department of Guidance and Counselling, Taraba State University, Jalingo, Nigeria

*Address all correspondence to: lucy.matsayi@tsuniversity.edu.ng

References

[1] Michlig GJ, Westergaard RP, Lam Y, Ahmadi A, Kirk GD, Genz A, et al. Avoidance, meaning and grief: Psychosocial factors influencing engagement in HIV care. AIDS Care. 2018;**30**(4):511-517. DOI: 10.1080/09540121.2018.1425366

[2] Shepherd A. Psychosocial meaning making in carceral spaces: A case study of prison and mental health care practice. Journal of Psychosocial Studies. 2021;**14**(2):139-151. DOI: 10.1332/147867321x16215933279607

[3] UNRWA. Psychosocial Support Recreational Activities Resource Guide. 2017. Retrieved from: https://www.unrwa.org/sites/default/files/content/resources/recreational_activities_resource_guide.pdf [Accessed: May 14, 2023]

[4] INEE. Education Sector Contingency Planning. 2018. Available from: http://www.ineesite.org/en/minimum-standards/contingency-planning [Accessed: May 14, 2023]

[5] Ekberg K, McDermott J, Moynihan C, Brindle L, Little P, Leydon GM. The role of helplines in cancer care: Intertwining emotional support with information or advice-seeking needs. Journal of Psychosocial Oncology. 2014;**32**(3):359-381. DOI: 10.1080/07347332.2014.897294

[6] Bell K. An exploration of Women's psychosocial support needs in the context of assisted reproduction. Social Work in Health Care. 2012;**51**(8):695-709. DOI: 10.1080/00981389.2012.696086

[7] Phibal A, Hatthakit U. Spiritual Care Needs and Spiritual Care Received. BMJ Supportive & Palliative Care. 2013;**3**(2):1-249. DOI: 10.1136/bmjspcare-2013-000491.62

[8] Nagaswami V. Integration of psychosocial rehabilitation in national health care programmes. Psychosocial Rehabilitation Journal. 1990;**14**(1):53-65. DOI: 10.1037/h0099455

[9] Parrish J. Supported housing: A critical component of effective community support. Psychosocial Rehabilitation Journal. 1990;**13**(4):9-10. DOI: 10.1037/h0099480

[10] Churchill R, Moore TH, Davies P, Caldwell D, Jones H, Lewis G, et al. Psychodynamic therapies versus other psychological therapies for depression. Cochrane Database of Systematic Reviews. 2010;(9):CD008706. DOI: 10.1002/14651858.CD008706. PMID: 25267905; PMCID: PMC4176678

[11] Perry D, Rubinstein D, Austin J. Animal-assisted group therapy in mental health settings: An initial model. Alternative and Complementary Therapies. 2012;**18**(4):181-185. DOI: 10.1089/act.2012.18403

[12] Thabrew H, Stasiak K, Hetrick SE, Donkin L, Huss JH, Highlander A, et al. Psychological therapies for anxiety and depression in children and adolescents with long-term physical conditions. Cochrane Database of Systematic Reviews. 2018;**12**(12):CD012488. DOI: 10.1002/14651858.CD012488.pub2. PMID: 30578633; PMCID: PMC6353208

[13] Rosenbaum P. Review: Some psychosocial interventions can help children and families cope with chronic health conditions. Evidence-Based Mental Health. 1998;**1**(2):48-48. DOI: 10.1136/ebmh.1.2.48

[14] Harrison J, Newell R, Small N. Do nurses' responses cause more distress than the presence of visions and voices? Mental Health Practice. 2008;**11**(5):17-19. DOI: 10.7748/mhp2008.02.11.5.17.c6339

[15] Trueland J. Common but crushing: How skin conditions can affect mental health. Nursing Standard. 2021;**36**(2):51-54. DOI: 10.7748/ns.36.2.51.s18

[16] Mindt MR, Spaulding WD. The coping strategies task: Assessment of coping in schizophrenia. Psychiatric Rehabilitation Skills. 2002;**6**(3):428-453. DOI: 10.1080/10973430208408446

[17] Dziegielewski SF. The coping skills program: Storybooks that teach cognitive, emotional and behavioral skills, by coping skills, LLC. Social Work in Mental Health. 2011;**9**(5):395-395. DOI: 10.1080/15332985.2011.576992

[18] Silverman MJ. Music-based affect regulation and unhealthy music use explain coping strategies in adults with mental health conditions. Community Mental Health Journal. 2020;**56**(5):939-946. DOI: 10.1007/s10597-020-00560-4

Section 3

Delivery of Treatment Services in Tertiary Care

Chapter 3

Delivery of Pharmaceutical Care at Tertiary Level: From Admission to Home Care

Nour Hanah Othman, Aina Amanina Abdul Jalil, Nor Safwan Hadi Nor Afendi and Syarifah Syamimi Putri Adiba Syed Putera

Abstract

Pharmaceutical care is a patient-centred practice that strives to optimise patients 'outcomes. In tertiary institutions, pharmaceutical care plays an important role in managing complex medical conditions and ensuring medication safety. Patients who attend tertiary care institutions are admitted for various reasons, and some of the conditions that warrant admissions are medication related. Patients, especially geriatrics may experience adverse reactions and drug interactions issues due to the multiple drugs that they consume. Some patients may have adherence issues that can lead to the worsening of their medical conditions. These pharmaceutical issues can be uncovered during their stay as inpatients through a thorough medication review. Pharmacists can play a role in providing knowledge and educating patients to overcome their medication-related problems. Monitoring of these problems can be undertaken through home visits by conducting home medication reviews, and other behavioural aspects of patient care, such as self-care, can be discovered.

Keywords: medication review, adverse drug reactions, medication adherence, home medication review, self-care

1. Introduction

1.1 Definition

The concept of pharmaceutical care (PC) emerged in the early 90's and has since evolved to become a recognised aspect of pharmacy practice. The philosophy of pharmaceutical care was introduced by Hepler and Strand in 1990 [1] and has been an important concept in every field of pharmacy practice in which patients are the focus. They have defined PC as 'the responsible provision of medical therapy for the purpose of achieving definite outcomes'. The process of pharmaceutical care involves pharmacists working with other healthcare professionals to develop, implement and monitor a therapeutic plan designed to produce specific therapeutic outcomes. These functions are carried out through a comprehensive assessment of the patient's health and drug history, devising, implementing appropriate plans of care, monitoring and evaluating the efficacy and safety of drug therapy.

The American Society of Hospital Pharmacists (ASHP), United States (US) is of the opinion that PC represents a valuable new concept representing growth in the profession beyond clinical pharmacy as often practiced. It also goes beyond pharmacists' activities, including medication preparation and dispensing. In 1992, ASHP came out with a new definition of PC, which is an adaptation of the definition developed by Hepler and Strand. ASHP defined pharmaceutical care as 'the direct responsible provision of medication-related care for the purpose of achieving definite outcomes that improve a patient's quality of life' [2]. The principal elements of PC by this definition are not only medication therapy but also decisions not to use medication therapy. The outcomes sought from PC are cure of a patient's disease, eradication, reduction in patients' symptoms, arresting or slowing of a patient's disease progression and prevention of a disease or symptoms.

The interest in the philosophy of PC is not only confined to the US where it was founded but also spread globally. While ASHP further elucidated the meaning of PC, the board of the Pharmaceutical Care Network Europe (PCNE) saw the need to redefine PC in 2013 for the purpose of having a single and certain definition in Europe. The redefinition reads 'pharmaceutical care is the pharmacist's contribution to the care of individuals in order to optimise medicines use and improve health outcomes' [3].

1.2 Pharmaceutical care at tertiary level care

PC is delivered through clinical pharmacy practice at primary, secondary and tertiary levels of care. With the ASHP PC definition that includes all medication-related problems, the practice has expanded, especially when it involves patients who are hospitalised. Pharmacists at tertiary care institutions incorporate pharmaceutical care through practices that include medication history-taking, drug regimen review and monitoring and reconciliation of medications.

Patients admitted at tertiary care centres are more critical due to the presence of co-morbidities and more drug-related problems that need urgent interventions. Studies have shown that there is a high prevalence of DRPs among patients who visited the emergency department or are admitted. An average of 1.25 (+1.23) drug-related problems (DRPs) per prescription was observed in chronic kidney disease patients. The most common DRP was adverse drug reactions [4]. Patients (N = 109) admitted to the emergency department observed for a period of 6 months were identified with various DRPs of which 69.7% was due to ADR, 27.5% non-adherence, followed by subtherapeutic doses, untreated indication and overdosage (0.91%) [5]. Pharmacists in tertiary care institutions work as part of a multidisciplinary healthcare team to provide pharmaceutical care services. They also ensure that the interventions are tailored to the unique needs of the patient and ensure treatment effectiveness and patient safety. Thus, the purpose of PC is to ensure that DRPs are discovered and recognised by pharmacists, so patients receive the right care for them to achieve definite outcomes and quality of life.

2. Medication review

2.1 Introduction

Medication review processes are changing in several countries as a result of pharmacists' increased involvement in drug history taking, medication reconciliation and medication review in their day-to-day work [6]. A medication review can be done independently or in tandem with other interventions such as medication reconciliation or personnel education. Although the clinical advantages of medication reviews, such as lowering hospital stay and mortality, have not always been demonstrated, medication management and multidisciplinary approaches have proven to be successful methods for reducing drug-related iatrogenic risks, inappropriate medication use and drug spending for elderly recipients [7].

An ageing population necessitates more medications and has a higher prevalence of multiple medical conditions. Age-related polypharmacy, which is the continuous use of five or more different medicines [8], is becoming more prevalent. There is ample proof that polypharmacy contributes to more problems with medication safety and a higher risk of adverse drug events (ADEs). The risk of drug interactions, drug toxicity, falls, delirium and non-adherence [9], as well as the possibility of readmission and mortality, have all been linked to polypharmacy [10]. The value of medication reviews by pharmacists for patients in community settings is becoming increasingly recognised through research [11]. The World Health Organisation (WHO) suggests giving patients who are taking numerous medications a medication review to lessen the risk of polypharmacy [12]. Medication reviews may lower the likelihood of polypharmacy, also known as the use of multiple medications, improper drug usage and medication costs in patients [13]. When a healthcare provider meets a patient and decides to prescribe or stop medication after going through an extensive and planned process that is supported by the patient's records, the process is known as a medication review [14]. The plan for discontinuing inappropriate therapy and achieving medication optimisation, therefore, incorporates a medication review [15].

It has been demonstrated that implementing a medication review effort, which allows identifying many underlying risk factors and coordinating explicit measures to lessen the effects of each can lower the incidence of inpatient falls by 20–30% [12]. Falls are a common and increasing concern to older people's both immediate and long-term health and functional independence [16]. In addition, falls are the most reported safety occurrence among adult inpatients [17]. A physical injury occurs in 30–50% of falls, and fractures happen in 1–3% of cases. Establishing effective fall prevention strategies, such as appropriate multifactorial interventions, is crucial due to the burden associated with fall injuries from both an individual and a societal standpoint. A medication review with the goal of carefully deprescribing certain medications is an essential component of a multifaceted approach to preventing falls [18].

2.2 Process

The requirement for criteria for competency has become clear as pharmacists' adoption of medication reviews has increased [19]. The criteria were developed based on Clyne et al.'s suggestion of three degrees of review comprehensiveness: prescription review, medication review and comprehensive medication review (CMR) [20].

The common medicine dispensing procedure includes an immediate review of the medication list known as a prescription for the medication. Whenever technical and therapeutic issues with the medication list may be resolved based on the information provided in the prescriptions, such as dosage and indication, they are considered in the prescription review.

Medication reviews, which evaluate the appropriateness of a prescription and identify and address therapeutically important medication-related issues, can be observed as a different service offered to the patient. It is advised that the medication review be carried out in a multidisciplinary setting along with the patient being informed of the drug of choice findings and adjustments. Checking proper medication use, adherence and self-management forms a component of medication review.

Compared to a medication review, a comprehensive medication review (CMR) is a more comprehensive assessment. Collaboration with the attending physician and other members of the care team will be utilised to address any clinically significant issues relating to the medication or medical condition. The patient is informed of significant medication observations and modifications. CMR involves ensuring that every medication is appropriate for consumption while considering the patient's illness and overall health. Upon CMRs, pharmacists collaborated with doctors and patients to manage medical conditions through patient education and motivational interviewing, medication adjustments and care coordination [21].

2.3 Importance

A medication review in combination with medication reconciliation, patient and professional education and transitional care is linked to a reduced chance of readmissions to the hospital [22]. Hospitalisations can have a negative impact on older patients' prognosis. Older patients are vulnerable to problems such as delirium, falls, functional degeneration, and future confinement or readmission following hospitalisation [23]. Readmissions due to medication are common, especially in elderly patients. Optimising medication appropriateness may lower medication-related issues and the frequency of hospital readmissions.

Medication reviews performed by clinical pharmacists' aid in the identification and prevention of medication errors and have been demonstrated to improve patient safety and reduce the risk of medication errors by up to 50% [24]. The annual incidence of preventable adverse drug events (ADEs) caused by medication errors in hospitalised patients is estimated to be 400,000 occurrences or approximately one medication error per patient each hospital day [25]. During all transitions of the hospital stay (admission, transfer of care, and discharge), the medication review process is described as verifying medication use, discovering discrepancies and resolving any medication-related difficulties [26].

Medication review by a clinical pharmacist can help older individuals with polypharmacy use their medications more effectively, especially when combined with cognitive functioning and depression screening [27]. Polypharmacy in the elderly commonly leads to medication therapy issues such as interactions, drug toxicity, falls with injury, delirium and non-adherence [9].

3. Medication reconciliation

3.1 Introduction

The report 'To Err Is Human' by the Institute of Medicine has highlighted medical errors as a substantial cause of patient harm [28]. The statistics on medical errors consistently present startling figures and are often alarming. A recent WHO report and Cochrane review indicate that during hospitalisation, specifically at the transition of care, a significant proportion of patients (ranging from 25 to 80%) encountered at least one medication discrepancy or experienced a failure to communicate changes in their medication regimen [29, 30]. In the context of the delivery of pharmaceutical care at the tertiary level, medication reconciliation is a pivotal measure that should be undertaken to ensure medication safety in the inpatient setting. Recently, the original concept of medication reconciliation has transformed resulting in the establishment of a patient-centred system that supports optimal medication management [31].

Medication reconciliation is a formalised and standardised process that entails cross-referencing the medications presently consumed by a patient with any newly prescribed medications at transitions of care such as admission, discharge or transfer with standard health care [32]. The primary objective of medication reconciliation is to identify and rectify any inadvertent discrepancies, omissions or duplications in medication orders, thereby fostering safe and accurate management of medications for the patient's well-being according to the standards of medication frequency, route, dose, combination and therapeutic purpose [33].

3.2 Process

Multiple initiatives are being implemented during patient care transitions to promote medication. Extensive measures have been adopted across all healthcare providers and several international patient safety organisations to guarantee the precise and consistent transfer of medication information for patients throughout the transition of care.

Medication reconciliation plays a vital role as a key service during care transitions and has been proven with remarkable effectiveness in mitigating potential medication error risks. National Institute for Health and Care Excellence (NICE) guidelines recommended medication reconciliation to be performed within 24 hours or earlier if deemed medically necessary within the transition of care [34].

In general, medicines reconciliation comprises three primary steps (**Figure 1**) [29].

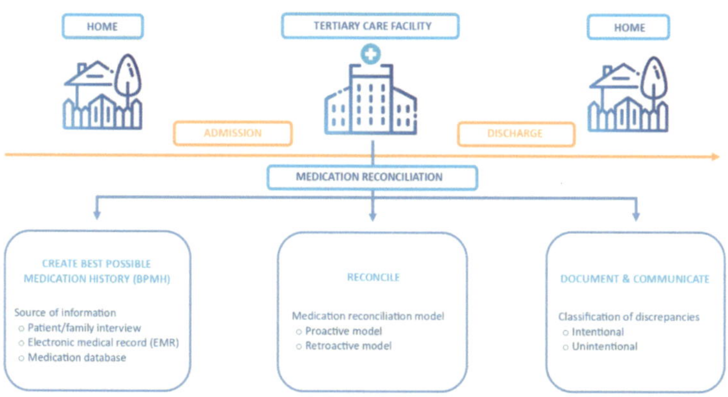

Figure 1.
Medication reconciliation process.

3.2.1 Creating the best possible medication history (BPMH)

At each juncture of care transitions, the identification of a patient's pre-transition medication regimen is paramount. BPMH is a comprehensive list of the current medications that a healthcare provider obtains from various sources of information prior to the care transition to capture essential medication information [31].

To gain this information, a systematic process is employed, ensuring that no critical information is overlooked. This process involves tapping into primary sources for obtaining an accurate medication history. The main sources for obtaining a medication history may include engaging in open and effective communication with the patient or their relatives. By accessing the electronic medical record (EMR) system within the institution, a wealth of up-to-date patient data, including medication profiles may also be obtained ensuring the completeness and accuracy of the BPMH. In addition, the medication profile provided by a third party can also serve as a valuable resource in the creation of BPMH [35].

By utilising these diverse sources of information, healthcare providers can piece together a comprehensive and accurate BPMH. This facilitates the seamless transition of medication information, promotes patient safety and optimises the quality of care provided during the care transition process. This step emphasises the significance of gathering accurate and up-to-date information regarding a patient's medication history to inform the subsequent medical decision-making process [36].

3.2.2 Comparing the BPMH with medicines prescribed on admission, at in-patient transfer or patient discharge and identifying discrepancies

During this crucial step, a comprehensive assessment is conducted for both prescribed and non-prescribed medications. Within the clinical context, two primary models, the proactive and retroactive models or a combination thereof can facilitate the medication reconciliation process [37].

In the proactive model, BPMH is established prior to formulating admission medication orders. By obtaining a comprehensive understanding of the patient's current medication regimen, potential drug interactions, allergies and other pertinent factors, healthcare providers can proactively address any discrepancies or potential risks to patient safety [38].

On the other hand, the retroactive model involves generating admission orders before creating the BPMH. Challenges in completing a BPMH due to delays in receiving the initial medication history from the prescriber in the retroactive model of medication reconciliation were particularly prominent in the critical care setting. Possible reasons for these delays included the challenges of approaching families during high-acuity situations and the lower priority given by physicians to medication reconciliation when engaged in acute patient care [39]. While this approach differs in sequence, it still necessitates a thorough reconciliation between the BPMH and the admission orders. This reconciliation step serves as a critical mechanism for identifying any disparities, inconsistencies or omissions that may exist between the documented medication history and the prescribed medications.

Regardless of any model employed, the reconciliation process bridged between the BPMH and the admission orders to ease the identification and rectification of any discrepancies. By comparing the patient's medication history with the prescribed medications, healthcare providers, such as pharmacists, can pinpoint potential issues such as drug interactions, duplicate therapies, incorrect dosages or the omission of crucial medications [40].

3.2.3 Reconciling discrepancies by classifying them as intentional or unintentional and by taking the appropriate action and documenting intervention

Once the discrepancies have been identified, they undergo a comprehensive and thorough analysis within the clinical context to ensure a detailed understanding of their nature and implications. This analysis allows for further classification of the discrepancies into two distinct categories: intentional and unintentional [41]. Intentional discrepancies arise from conscious decisions made by either the patient or the healthcare provider such as intentional adjustments to the medication regimen based on specific considerations. In contrast, unintentional discrepancies encompass instances where changes in the medication history occur without a conscious decision being made. These can manifest as both omission errors, where a medication is unintentionally left out or not properly documented and commission errors, where a medication is unintentionally added or administered incorrectly. Paediatric patients are a highly vulnerable population identified with unintentional discrepancies during the transition of care [42].

4. Home medication review

4.1 Introduction

4.1.1 Importance of medication management at home

Many patients are hospitalised for chronic conditions such as hypertension, diabetes, asthma, arthritis and cardiovascular diseases, especially geriatrics. As a result, they are given multiple types of medications and polypharmacy is common. There are various drug-related problems (DRPs) that can arise because of polypharmacy such as drug-drug interactions, adverse drug reactions (ADRs), medication errors and drug-food interactions, which may have a detrimental effect on medication adherence [43]. Patients may also forget to take their medications, alter the dose or frequency of their medications or discontinue their medications. Thus, inappropriate medication use among patients is a major health concern, especially among vulnerable patients such as geriatrics [44] and psychiatric patients [45]. ADRs are DRPs that are a major burden to patients, as shown by the fact it is the highest DRP found at admission [4, 5]. Therefore, to address these DRPs at home, home medication review (HMR) was first initiated in Australia [46] and followed by many other countries [45].

4.1.2 Purpose and scope of home medication review

The purpose of HMR is to assist in identifying, addressing medication-related problems and optimising medication regimens. An accredited pharmacist will conduct the medication review to help people to better understand how to manage their medicines and minimise adverse drug events [47].

4.2 Understanding home medicines review

4.2.1 Definition and objectives

HMR is a process designed to ensure that patients take their medicines correctly at home so that medications are used safely and effectively [48]. The term home medication review is also used interchangeably and has the same definition and process as HMR.

4.2.2 Healthcare professionals' roles

An HMR is intended for the patient's to gain maximum benefit from their medication regimen and prevent medication-related problems through a team approach. This is achieved by conducting a home visit by the healthcare professional team consisting of doctors, nurses and pharmacists and involving the carers.

HMR involves the pharmacist responsibility to assess the patient's adherence to their medications, identify any issues related to the patient's medication regimen and empower the patient and caregiver's knowledge of their disease. They also make recommendations on patients' treatment plans to the responsible health practitioner. This helps to increase the quality use of medicines and decrease adverse events.

Applying HMR to discharged patients is a vital tool to ensure that patients receive proper care and management of their medications during the transition of care. The continuum of quality use of medicines between hospitals and the community needs to be maintained [49]. In the formal process of continuity of care between the hospital and the community, a liaison pharmacist will organise an appointment post-discharge. He/she will contact the community pharmacist to engage an accredited pharmacist to carry out the HMR, as well as to arrange for the report to be sent to the general practitioner and the community pharmacist.

HMR applies to many types of conditions. The three most common types of HMR are HMR Neurology/Stroke, HMR Psychiatry and HMR Geriatrics. However, patients with other chronic conditions may also require the HMR service depending on the assessments made on them.

4.3 The HMR process

An accredited pharmacist HMR clinical process is categorised into three stages: [50].

Stage 1: Information gathering and review.

The HMR process begins with a referral from the doctor (hospital, GP or CP). The initial assessment will include the reason for referral and the patient's medical and medication history. The pharmacist will conduct a thorough review of the patient's medication including prescription, over-the-counter and complementary medicine.

Stage 2: Pharmacist consultation.

The pharmacist will conduct a face-to-face consultation with the patient and his/her carer. The medications will be carefully reviewed to identify any potential issues such as drug interactions, duplications, incorrect dosages or medications that are no longer necessary. The pharmacist will assess the person's understanding of their medications, including how and when to take them, any potential side effects and the purpose of each medication.

Stage 3: HMR documentation.

This is the stage whereby the accredited pharmacist collates, generates, prepares the findings and recommends interventions. The complete report will be given to the referring doctor for his consideration to optimise prescribing, enhance patient management and optimise patient's health.

4.4 Benefits and outcomes

The value of HMR has been shown by two studies related to older adults and under-served groups. Frail and homebound community-dwelling geriatrics were observed to be using a high number of medications and experiencing a significant number of

DRPs. Recommendations to optimise medication therapy by community pharmacists can be effectively done by HMR [51]. Likewise, underserved communities in Taiwan had many issues with medications, but with pharmacists' home visits, their knowledge of diseases improved and drug-related problems were mitigated, while drug compliance and drug storage methods were improved resulting in less drug wastage [52].

The program *managing your blood pressure* was implemented in a cohort of geriatric African Americans with hypertension to reduce health disparities in blood pressure control. The percentage of patients with controlled BP increased from 46.7% to 49.5%. All other parameters, including knowledge of hypertension, medication adherence and self-monitoring of BP improved significantly from baseline to post-intervention [53]. The positive effect of HMR on psychiatric patients was shown by a study in which the impact of a hospital pharmacist-led home medication review programme on 133 patients with schizophrenia. The patients showed significant improvement in medication adherence, knowledge of antipsychotic drugs and quality of life on social and family components [45].

A retrospective review of HMR cases was performed on 224 community-dwelling older people (65 years or older). Most of the pharmacists' recommended actions during the medication review process were consistent with the literature embedded in key Australian information sources. Medication management in older people is complex and challenging as the DRPs identified were 98%. In this vulnerable population, a pharmacist with appropriate training and access to the patient's medical record can assist with improving the quality of medication use [54].

HMR has become an accepted service in many countries as pharmacist-led medicines review has been shown to improve health outcomes [45, 52, 53]. However, there are limited studies that have investigated the cost-effectiveness of HMR by accredited pharmacists. Rosli et al. evaluated the cost-effectiveness of home medication review by community pharmacists and found that it is a cost-effective option that significantly reduced HbA1c levels among T2DM patients, although it was associated with higher mean total costs per participant [55]. This suggests that home medication review programs such as HMR-CP could minimise patients' health-related costs and burdens, thereby enhancing the quality of life and well-being. More economic analyses and cost-effectiveness studies are needed to find evidence of the economic benefits of HMR.

5. Medication-related problems (MRP)

5.1 Introduction

The pharmaceutical profession has evolved beyond traditional roles such as drug formulation and dispensing into a highly regulated profession focused on individualised and direct patient care [56]. Medication-related problems (MRP) are a common but preventable problem in healthcare. It is defined as 'an event or circumstance related to drug therapy that actually or potentially interferes with desired health outcomes' [57]. A medication-related problem (MRP) is a suboptimal situation in which a particular treatment regimen is likely to produce or contribute to an undesirable outcome [58].

In our daily lives, various populations simply or implicitly rely on medications to prevent and treat infections and lifelong MRPs occur in any period of drug use. They can appear after as short as an hour of medication consumption [59]. The World Health Organisation (WHO) estimates that more than half of all medicines are prescribed, dispensed or sold improperly, and more than one-half of patients do not take them correctly [60]. Previous study stipulates that pharmacists help improve drug therapy and optimise outcomes by recognising, avoiding and resolving MRPs [61]. Hospitalisations, unnecessary clinic visits and prolonged care can be caused by unresolved or latent MRPs, which not only impede clinical treatment but also increases the financial burden for patients [62]. Often, MRPs can be related to an error in drug treatment (medication error), or they can be caused by a medication side effect (adverse drug reaction) [63]. Factors such as mismanagement, population growth, poor health systems and lack of primary health care research and evaluation have limited the development of primary health care [64].

Early intervention and containment of MRPs can significantly reduce physician visits, emergency room visits, hospitalisations and healthcare costs while improving overall patient health and quality of life [65].

5.2 Medication history assessment

Upon admission to the hospital, a medication history assessment is performed to obtain and document a complete list of the patient's medication history. This includes prescription and over-the-counter medicines, dietary supplements and traditional medicines [66]. Drug histories are often incomplete, drug strengths, frequency, dosages and forms are missing, and complementary or over-the-counter (OTC) medications are often taken out. Previous studies have shown that 10–67% of drug histories contain at least one error [67]. Incorrect medication history can lead to treatment interruptions, reintroduction of discontinued medications, inappropriate treatment and undetected drug-related problems. The continuation of these errors upon discharge can lead to adverse events due to duplication of treatment, drug interactions and discontinuation of an essential medication [68]. Additional information, such as treatment adherence and past allergy or anaphylaxis and adverse reactions, should be recorded and compared to the patient's previous medical or hospital admission records [69].

A previous study in Malaysia found that 990 treatment discrepancies were identified in 390 patients recruited from three general medicine departments at Sarawak General Hospital. Of these, 135 (13.6%) medical errors were identified in 93 (23.8%) patients (1.45 errors per patient), most of which were due to medication omissions (79%) [70]. Similarly, it was found that the majority (83%) of 168 patients admitted to two gastrointestinal surgery wards and one geriatric ward at St. Olav's University Hospital in Trondheim and two general internal medicine wards at Ålesund Hospital, Norway for a period of 3 months had at least one drug discrepancy in their medical history. Drug omissions accounted for 72% of the discrepancies, while dose differences accounted for the remaining 28%. A total of 9% of the disparity could have caused serious damage or inconvenience [71].

5.3 Prescribing medicines

When there is a change in care, errors in a patient's treatment plan can occur, particularly during a hospital stay, a transfer from an emergency room to another department or intensive care unit (ICU), a transfer from an ICU or from an operating room to a ward and a transfer from the hospital to home or to another facility, such as a nursing home [68]. Previous studies found that 30%–70% were unintentional discrepancies between the medications patients were taking before admission and their prescriptions at admission [72]. In a recent study, 26.6% of these discrepancies were due to insufficient or incorrect information on primary care medication lists, including primary care referrals and medication printouts [73].

The lack of a drug with a valid indication is the most common unintentional discrepancy, and about half of these errors can go unnoticed before impacting the patient [74]. Discrepancies during discharge often arise when prescriptions are being made and discharge notes are drawn up. An Australian study found that 15% of medications that should have been continued were omitted from the discharge prescription [75]. Another study found that 12% of patients made one or more errors in the prescriptions, including accidental omissions and discontinuation of subsequent medications [76]. Patients who forgot one or more medications on their discharge report are 2.31 times more likely than usual to be hospitalised [77].

MRPs are very common in the prescribing phase, especially in the emergency department (ED) [78]. It is estimated that at least 3% of all hospital-related adverse drug reactions occur in ED as it is among the most sought department, which offers a 24-hour medical care service [79]. A previous study conducted in the ED of a United States (US) tertiary hospital found that nearly 54% of MRPs occurred during the prescribing phase [80]. Another study conducted at a tertiary hospital in India found that MRPs are present in 16.2% of ED prescriptions [81].

A review has found that incorrect dosage, frequency and strength were the most common prescribing errors [82]. A previous systematic review of 50 published studies, mainly from Iran, Saudi Arabia, Egypt and Jordan, found that the most common factors contributing to the prescribing errors in these studies were lack of knowledge, understaffing and heavy workload [83].

Previous studies have documented the rates of prescribing errors in Australia's various acute care settings whereby insights into prescription error rates were explained when different prescribing systems (traditional and electronic) are used [84–86]. Taken together, these studies found that prescribing errors were more prominent in traditional or paper-based systems in hospitals, there were roughly about five errors per patient. Nonetheless, these mainly involve errors in the documentation such as unclear handwriting or prescriptions, missing signatures and missing routes of administration [87]. A slightly lower error rate was reported when using the standardised medical record. Some studies also found that the overall rate of typos with electronic writing systems is half of the traditional system, with about two per admission [86, 87].

5.4 Medication administration

In a previous review that looked into drug safety in critical care, it was found that medication errors varied depending on the type of system used. After excluding timing errors, they found that the rate of administration errors such as removal of therapy and incorrect dosing ranged from 5 to 8% when individualised patient delivery systems were used, and from 15to 18% when ward stock systems were in charge [88].

It was found that approximately 9% of drug administrations were associated with clinical errors (excluding timing errors) at two main teaching hospitals in New South Wales, Australia. This study also examined how the error rate changed with intrusions and disturbances during drug administration where at each occurrence, the probability of procedural and clinical errors increased by 12% and 13%, respectively [89].

Meanwhile, in an observational study involving intravenous (IV) drug administration, incorrect infusion rates accounted for 95 of the 101 major errors and bolus administration was more likely to be associated with more serious errors (23% vs. 10.6% for other IV routes). Infusion pump error rates were similar to other methods [90].

6. Self-care

6.1 Introduction

6.1.1 What is self-care?

The WHO has defined self-care as 'the ability of individuals, families and communities to promote health, prevent disease, maintain health and cope with illness and disability with or without the support of a healthcare provider' [91].

The practice of self-care empowers people to take charge of their health and well-being, giving them the incentive to live a healthier and happier life. It is key to preventing certain conditions and improving recovery times when total prevention fails. In every stage of life, it is an essential part of well-being [92].

Self-care involved: [92].

a. Making healthy lifestyle choices such as eating healthy food, exercising and work-life balance.

b. Avoiding unhealthy lifestyle habits such as smoking, vaping and drinking alcohol.

c. Making responsible use of prescription and non-prescription items. This includes avoiding abusing addictive substances.

d. Self-recognition of symptoms and assessing and addressing symptoms in collaboration with healthcare providers, when necessary.

e. Self-monitoring of own conditions to check for signs of deterioration or improvement and knowing when to get professional help.

f. Self-managing symptoms of disease, either alone, with carers or in partnership with healthcare professionals.

6.1.2 Importance of self-care

The importance of self-care lies in the empowerment of people to take control of their health and well-being and to improve their quality of life for the better [92]. Self-care can help certain conditions and improve recovery times when total prevention does not work. In all stages of life, it is an integral part of well-being. As people's life expectancy continues to rise globally, there has been a proportional increase in the number of individuals living with chronic conditions [93]. This circumstance has prompted individuals to autonomously manage and seamlessly incorporate their health conditions into their daily routine [94]. To be able to manage this situation well, healthy individuals or those living with chronic conditions need to know how to conduct it. The achievement of effective self-care necessitates a proactive collaboration between consumers and healthcare providers (HCPs), including pharmacists, and is contingent upon well informed consumers and HCPs equipped with proficient communication abilities [95].

Upon discharge from the hospital, patients encounter a multitude of challenges. This transitional phase places patients at risk of unnecessary harm due to insufficient preparation before their discharge, thereby potentially giving rise to errors and compromising their well-being [96]. It is during the discharge phase that proper medication reconciliation and comprehensive education sessions between pharmacists and patients, and their caregivers should take place to prepare patients for self-care while at home.

There is the potential for substantial healthcare cost savings from enhancing the self-care options that are available to consumers. It was estimated that 10–25% of GP consultations in different European countries could be substituted by self-care, which varies from country to country, depending on the current level of self-care uptake. Further substitution of GP visits by responsible self-care could release 17.6 billion euros per year for society [97].

7. Conclusions

Collaboration between healthcare providers, including pharmacists and well informed consumers is essential when it comes to managing medical conditions at the tertiary level. This is important to ensure that patients get the best possible care starting from admission to discharge. The practice of self-care can bring significant advantages to individuals and society by relieving the burden on medical resources. Pharmacists have a crucial role to play in ensuring proper medication management and continuity of care encompassing activities such as home medicines review (HMR) and discharge planning. Maintaining a seamless continuum of quality medicine use from hospitals to the community is paramount in guaranteeing patients receive the appropriate level of care.

Conflict of interest

The authors declare no conflict of interest.

Author details

Nour Hanah Othman*, Aina Amanina Abdul Jalil, Nor Safwan Hadi Nor Afendi and Syarifah Syamimi Putri Adiba Syed Putera
Universiti Kuala Lumpur Royal College of Medicine Perak, Malaysia

*Address all correspondence to: nourhanah@unikl.edu.my

References

[1] Hepler CD, Strand LM. Opportunities and responsibilities in pharmaceutical care. American Journal of Hospital Pharmacy. 1990;**47**(3):533-543

[2] American Society of Health System Pharmacy. ASHP statement on pharmaceutical care. American Journal of Hospital Pharmacy. 1993;**50**:1720-1723. Available from: https://www.ashp.org/pharmacy-practice/policy-positions-and-guidelines/browser-by-document-type/statements [Accessed: May 23, 2023]

[3] Allemann SS, van Mil JW, Botermann L, Berger K, Griese N, Hersberger KE. Pharmaceutical care: The PCNE definition 2013. International Journal of Clinical Pharmacy. 2014;**36**(3):544-555. DOI: 10.1007/s11096-014-9933-x

[4] Sakthirajan R, Varghese S, Roshni S, Sai LP, Muhammed SMJ, Ramalakshmi S. Identification of drug related problems among chronic disease patients in a tertiary care hospital. Saudi Journal of Medical and Pharmaceutical Sciences. 2019;**5**(11):949-955

[5] Akshay TL, Prakash A, Anas MAM, Diwaha S, Rama P. A prospective observational study on the incidence of drug-related hospital admissions in a tertiary care hospital. Asian Journal of Pharmaceutical and Clinical Research. 2021;**14**(4):56-59

[6] Leikola S, Tuomainen L, Peura S, Laurikainen A, Lyles A, Savela E, et al. Comprehensive medication review: Development of a collaborative procedure. International Journal of Clinical Pharmacy. 2012;**34**(4):510-514. DOI: 10.1007/s11096-012-9662-y

[7] Lee SWH, Mak VSL, Tang YW. Pharmacist services in nursing homes: A systematic review and meta-analysis. British Journal of Clinical Pharmacology. 2019;**85**(12):2668-2688. DOI: 10.1111/bcp.14101

[8] Masnoon N, Shakib S, Kalisch-Ellett L, Caughey GE. What is polypharmacy? A systematic review of definitions. BMC Geriatrics. 2017;**17**(1):230. DOI: 10.1186/s12877-017-0621-2

[9] Hoel RW, Giddings Connolly RM, Takahashi PY. Polypharmacy management in older patients. Mayo Clinic Proceedings. 2021;**96**(1):242-256. DOI: 10.1016/j.mayocp.2020.06.012

[10] Hilmer SN, Gnjidic D. The effects of polypharmacy in older adults. Clinical Pharmacology and Therapeutics. 2009;**85**(1):86-88. DOI: 10.1038/clpt.2008.224

[11] Midão L, Giardini A, Menditto E, Kardas P, Costa E. Polypharmacy prevalence among older adults based on the survey of health, ageing and retirement in Europe. Archives of Gerontology and Geriatrics. 2018;**78**:213-220. DOI: 10.1016/j.archger.2018.06.018

[12] Alpana MAIR. Medication Safety in Polypharmacy. Geneva: World Health Organization; 2019;(WHO/UHC/SDS/2019.11). Licence: CC BY-NC-SA 3.0 IGO

[13] Chen TF. Pharmacist-led home medicines review and residential medication management review: The Australian model. Drugs & Aging. 2016;**33**(3):199-204. DOI: 10.1007/s40266-016-0357-2

[14] National Institute for Health and Care Excellence (NICE). Medicines

Optimisation: The Safe and Effective Use of Medicines to Enable the Best Possible Outcomes. 2023: Available from: www.nice.org.uk/guidance/ng5

[15] Silva R de OS, Macêdo LA, GADJ S, Aguiar PM, De Lyra DPJ. Pharmacist-participated medication review in different practice settings: Service or intervention? An overview of systematic reviews. PLoS One. 2019;**14**(1):e0210312. DOI: 10.1371/journal.pone.0210312

[16] Montero-Odasso M, Van der Velde N, Alexander NB, Becker C, Blain H, Camicioli R, et al. New horizons in falls prevention and management for older adults: A global initiative. Age and Ageing. 2021;**50**(5):1499-1507. DOI: 10.1093/ageing/afab076

[17] Morris R, O'Riordan S. Prevention of falls in hospital. Clinical Medicine (London, England). 2017;**17**(4):360-362. DOI: 10.7861/clinmedicine.17-4-360

[18] Hopewell S, Adedire O, Copsey BJ, Boniface GJ, Sherrington C, Clemson L, et al. Multifactorial and multiple component interventions for preventing falls in older people living in the community. The Cochrane Database of Systematic Reviews. 2018;7(7):CD012221. DOI: 10.1002/14651858.CD012221.pub2

[19] Competency N, Framework S, Pharmacists FOR. National Competency Standards Framework for Pharmacists in Australia. Australia: National Policy Unit Pharmaceutical Society of Australia; 2016

[20] Clyne W, Blenkinsopp A SR. A guide to medication review. NPC Plus and Medicines Partnership. 2008. Available from: https://www.google.com/search?q=a+guide+to+medication+review&oq=a+guide+to+medication+review&aqs=chrome.69i57j35i39j0l3j69i64.8381j0j7&sourceid=chrome&ie=UTF-8

[21] Salvo MC, Cannon-Breland ML. Motivational interviewing for medication adherence. In: Journal of the American Pharmacists Association. United Sates: American Pharmacists Association; 2015;**55**(4):e354-e363. DOI: 10.1331/JAPhA.2015.15532

[22] Dautzenberg L, Bretagne L, Koek HL, Tsokani S, Zevgiti S, Rodondi N, et al. Medication review interventions to reduce hospital readmissions in older people. Journal of the American Geriatrics Society. 2021;**69**(6):1646-1658. DOI: 10.1111/jgs.17041

[23] Szlejf C, Farfel JM, Curiati JA, de BJ CE, Jacob-Filho W, Azevedo RS. Medical adverse events in elderly hospitalized patients: A prospective study. Clinics (Sao Paulo, Brazil). 2012;**67**(11):1247-1252. DOI: 10.6061/clinics/2012(11)04

[24] Jaam M, Naseralallah LM, Hussain TA, Pawluk SA. Pharmacist-led educational interventions provided to healthcare providers to reduce medication errors: A systematic review and meta-analysis. PLoS One. 2021;**16**(6):e0253588. DOI: 10.1371/journal.pone.0253588

[25] Bates DW. Preventing medication errors: A summary. American Journal of Health-System Pharmacy: AJHP: Official Journal of the American Society of Health-System Pharmacists. 2007;**64**(14 Suppl 9):S3-S9. DOI: 10.2146/ajhp070190

[26] Mertens V, Jacobs L, Knops N, Alemzadeh SM, Vandeven K, Swartenbroekx J, et al. Bedside medication review with cognitive and depression screening by a clinical pharmacist as part of a comprehensive geriatric assessment in hospitalized older patients with

polypharmacy: A pilot study. PLoS One. 2022;**17**(10):e0276402. DOI: 10.1371/journal.pone.0276402

[27] Agrawal A, Wu WY. Reducing medication errors and improving systems reliability using an electronic medication reconciliation system. Joint Commission Journal on Quality and Patient Safety. 2009;**35**(2):106-114. DOI: 10.1016/s1553-7250(09)35014-x

[28] Institute of Medicine (US). In: Kohn LT, Corrigan JM, Donaldson MS, editors. Committee on Quality of Health Care in America. To Err Is Human: Building a Safer Health System. Washington (DC): National Academies Press (US); 2000

[29] World Health Organization. Medication Safety in Transitions of Care. Geneva: World Health Organization; 2019. p. 50. WHO/UHC/SDS/2019.9. Licence: CC BY-NC-SA 3.0 IGO

[30] Redmond P, Grimes TC, McDonnell R, Boland F, Hughes C, Fahey T. Impact of medication reconciliation for improving transitions of care. Cochrane Database of Systematic Reviews. 2018;**8**(8):CD010791. DOI: 10.1002/14651858.CD010791.pub2

[31] Fernandes O. Medication reconciliation in the hospital: What, why, where, when, who and how? Healthcare Quarterly. 2012:42-49. DOI: 10.12927/hcq.2012.22842

[32] World Health Organization. Medication Safety in Polypharmacy. Geneva: World Health Organization; 2019. p. 61. WHO/UHC/SDS/2019.11. Licence: CC BY-NC-SA 3.0 IGO

[33] International Pharmaceutical Federation (FIP). Medication review and medicines use review: A toolkit for pharmacists. 2nd ed. The Hague: International Pharmaceutical Federation; 2022:29

[34] NICE Medicines and Prescribing Centre (UK). Medicines Optimisation: The Safe and Effective Use of Medicines to Enable the Best Possible Outcomes. Manchester: National Institute for Health and Care Excellence (NICE); 2015

[35] Chen HH, Taylor SE, Harding AM, Taylor DM. Accuracy of medication information sources compared to the best possible medication history for patients presenting to the emergency department. Emergency Medicine Australasia. 2018;**30**(5):654-661. DOI: 10.1111/1742-6723.12965

[36] Huang PP, Poon SY, Chang SH, Kuo CW, Chien MW, Chen CC, et al. Improving the efficiency of medication reconciliation in two Taiwanese hospitals by using the Taiwan National Health Insurance PharmaCloud medication system. International Journal of General Medicine. 2023;**16**:211-220. DOI: 10.2147/IJGM.S389683

[37] World Health Organization. High 5s Project Standard Operating Protocol. Assuring Accuracy of Medication Information at Transitions in Care: Medication Reconciliation. Geneva: World Health Organization; 2014. p. 36

[38] Leguelinel-Blache G, Arnaud F, Bouvet S, Dubois F, Castelli C, Roux-Marson C, et al. Impact of admission medication reconciliation performed by clinical pharmacists on medication safety. European Journal of Internal Medicine. 2014;**25**(9):808-814. DOI: 10.1016/j.ejim.2014.09.012

[39] Chan C, Woo R, Seto W, Pong S, Gilhooly T, Russell J. Medication reconciliation in pediatric cardiology performed by a pharmacy technician: A prospective cohort comparison study. The Canadian Journal of Hospital Pharmacy. 2015;**68**(1):8-15. DOI: 10.4212/cjhp.v68i1.1419

[40] Canning ML, Munns A, Tai B. Accuracy of best possible medication history documentation by pharmacists at an Australian tertiary referral metropolitan hospital. European Journal of Hospital Pharmacy. 2018;**25**(e1):e52-e58. DOI: 10.1136/ejhpharm-2016-001177

[41] Kwan JL, Lo L, Sampson M, Shojania KG. Medication reconciliation during transitions of care as a patient safety strategy: A systematic review. Annals of Internal Medicine. 2013;**158**(5 Pt 2):397-403. DOI: 10.7326/0003-4819-158-5-201303051-00006

[42] Abu Farha R, Abu Hammour K, Al-Jamei S, AlQudah R, Zawiah M. The prevalence and clinical seriousness of medication discrepancies identified upon hospital admission of pediatric patients. BMC Health Services Research. 2018;**18**(1):966. DOI: 10.1186/s12913-018-3795-1

[43] Hajjar ER, Cafiero AC, Hanlon JT. Polypharmacy in elderly patients. The American Journal of Geriatric Pharmacotherapy. 2007;**5**:345-351

[44] Castelino RL, Bajorek BV, Chen TF. Retrospective evaluation of home medicines review by pharmacists in older Australian patients using the medication appropriateness index. The Annals of Pharmacotherapy. 2010;**44**:1922-1929

[45] Tan YM, Chong CP, Chong YC. Impact of hospital pharmacist-led home medication review program for people with schizophrenia: A prospective study from Malaysia. Journal of Applied Pharmaceutical Science. 2019;**9**(07):034-041

[46] Ahn J, Park JE, Anthony C, Burke M. Understanding, Benefits, and Difficulties of Home Medicines Review. Available from https://www.racpg.org.au/afp/2015/apr/understanding-benefits-difficulties-of-home-me

[47] Home Medicines Review. Available from: https://www.ppaonline.com.au/programs/medication-management-pograms/home-medicines-review

[48] Home Medicines Review. Available from: https://healthdirect.gov.au/home-medicines-review

[49] Yu K, Nguyen A, Shakib S, Doecke CJ, Boyce M, March G, et al. Enhancing continuity of care in therapeutics: Development of a post-discharge home medicines review model. Journal of Pharmacy Practice and Research. 2015;**37**(1):22-26

[50] Patounas M, Lau ET, Chan V, Rigby D, Kyle GJ, Khatri J, et al. Home medicines review: A national survey of Australian accredited pharmacists' health service time investment. Pharmacy Practice (Granada). 2021;**19**(3):2376

[51] Lin W, Haq S, Sinha S, Fan-Lun C. Impact analysis of a pharmacist-led home-medication review service within an interprofessional outreach team. The Senior Care Pharmacist. 2021;**36**(3):159-170

[52] Lian YH, Wang KH, Huang HM, Shia BC, Chan SY, Ho CW, et al. Reducing medication problems among minority individuals with low socioeconomic status through pharmacist home visits. International Journal of Environmental Research and Public Health. 2022;**19**:4234

[53] Moultry AM, Pounds K, Poon IO. Managing medication adherence in elderly hypertensive patients through pharmacist home visits. The Consultant Pharmacist. 2015;**30**(12):710-719

[54] Castelino RL, Bajorek BV, Chen TF. Are interventons recommended by pharmacists during home medicines review evidence-based? Journal of Evaluation in Clinical Practice. 2011;**17**(1):104-110

[55] Rosli MR, Wu DBC, Neo CF, Karuppannan M. Economic evaluation of home medication review by community pharmacists (HMR-CP) for patients with type 2 diabetes mellitus (T2DM). Journal of Medical Economics. 2021;**24**(1):730-740

[56] Langebrake C, Hilgarth H. Clinical pharmacists' interventions in a German university hospital. Pharmacy World & Science. 2010;**32**(2):194-199. DOI: 10.1007/s11096-010-9367-z

[57] Thomsen LA,Winterstein AG, Søndergaard B, Haugbølle LS, Melander A. Systematic review of the incidence and characteristics of preventable adverse drug events in ambulatory care. Annals of Pharmacotherapy. 2007;**41**(9):1411-1426. DOI: 10.1345/aph.1H658

[58] Banks DL, Amin NS, Bardolia C, Awadalla MS, Knowlton CH, Bain KT. Medication-related problems encountered in the program of all-inclusive Care for the Elderly: An observational study. Journal of the American Pharmacists Association. 2020;**60**(2):319-327. DOI: 10.1016/j.japh.2019.10.012

[59] Augustine DV, Nambiar DP, Saseendran M, Anshila MK, Siva S. A review on drug related problems in a tertiary care teaching hospital, India. International Journal of Research and Review. 2020;**7**(5):270-276

[60] Plácido AI, Herdeiro MT, Morgado M, Figueiras A, Roque F. Drug-related problems in home-dwelling older adults: A systematic review. Clinical Therapeutics. 2020;**42**(4):559-572. DOI: 10.1016/j.clinthera.2020.02.005

[61] Isetts BJ, Buffington DE, Carter BL, Smith M, Polgreen LA, James PA. Evaluation of pharmacists' work in a physician-pharmacist collaborative model for the management of hypertension. Pharmacotherapy. 2016;**36**(4):374-384. DOI: 10.1016/j.japh.2019.10.012

[62] Ni XF, Yang CS, Bai YM, Hu ZX, Zhang LL. Drug-related problems of patients in primary health care institutions: A systematic review. Frontiers in Pharmacology. 2021;**12**:698907. DOI: 10.3389/fphar.2021.698907

[63] van den Bemt PMLA, Egberts TCG, Jong-Van D, den Berg LTW, Brouwers JRBJ. Drug-related problems in hospitalised patients. Drug Safety. 2012;**22**:321-333. DOI: 10.2165/00002018-200022040-00005

[64] Walley J, Lawn JE, Tinker A, de Francisco A, Chopra M, Rudan I, et al. Primary health care: Making Alma-Ata a reality. The Lancet. 2008;**372**(9642):1001-1007. DOI: 10.1016/S0140-6736(08)61409-9

[65] Rogan EL, Ranson CA, Valle-Oseguera CS, Lee C, Gumberg A, Nagin BN, et al. Factors associated with medication related problems in an ambulatory medicare population and the case for medication therapy management. Research in Social and Administrative Pharmacy. 2020;**16**(6):783-786. DOI: 10.1016/j.sapharm.2019.08.033

[66] The Joint Commission. Medication Reconciliation. Sentinel Event Alert, Issue 35. Updated January 25, 2006. Available from: http://www.jointcommission.org/SentinelEvents/

SentinelEventAlert/sea_35.htm [Accessed: May 26, 2023]

[67] Vira T, Colquhoun M, Etchells EE. Reconcilable differences: Correcting medication errors at hospital admission and discharge. Quality and Safety in Health Care. 2006;**15**(2):122-126. DOI: 10.1136/qshc.2005.015347

[68] Duguid M. The importance of medication reconciliation for patients and practitioners. Australian Prescriber. 2012;**35**:15-19. DOI: 10.18773/austprescr.2012.007

[69] Shenfield GM, Robb T, Duguid M. Recording previous adverse drug reactions – A gap in the system. British Journal of Clinical Pharmacology. 2001;**51**(6):623-626. DOI: 10.1111/j.1365-2125.2001.01380.x

[70] Oh AL, Tan AGHK, Chieng IYY. Detection of medication errors through medication history assessment during admission at general medical wards. Journal of Pharmacy Practice. 2022;**35**(3):407-412. DOI: 10.1177/0897190020987127

[71] Sund JK, Sletvold O, Mellingsæter TC, et al. Discrepancies in drug histories at admission to gastrointestinal surgery, internal medicine and geriatric hospital wards in Central Norway: A cross-sectional study. BMJ Open. 2017;**7**(9):e013427. DOI: 10.1136/bmjopen-2016-013427

[72] National Institute for Health and Clinical Excellence and National Patient Safety Agency. Technical Patient Safety Solutions for Medicines Reconciliation on Admission of Adults to Hospital. London: NHS; 2007

[73] Green CF, Burgul K, Armstrong DJ. A study of the use of medicine lists in medicines reconciliation: Please remember this, a list is just a list. International Journal of Pharmacy Practice. 2010;**18**(2):116-121

[74] Santell JP. Reconciliation failures lead to medication errors. The Joint Commission Journal on Quality and Patientient Safety. 2006;**32**(4):225-229. DOI: 10.1016/s1553-7250(06)32029-6

[75] Coombes ID, Storie WJ, Radford JM, Pillans PI. Quality of medication ordering at a large teaching hospital. The Australian Journal of Hospital Pharmacy. 2001;**31**(2):102-106. DOI: 10.1002/jppr2001312102

[76] Duguid M, Gibson M, O'Doherty R. Review of discharge prescriptions by pharmacists integral to continuity of care. Journal of Pharmacy Practice and Research. 2002;**32**(2):94-95

[77] Stowasser D, Collins D, Stowasser M. A randomised controlled trial of medication liaison services - Patient outcomes. Journal of Pharmacy Practice and Research. 2002;**32**(2):133-140. DOI: 10.1002/jppr2002322133

[78] Weant KA, Bailey AM, Baker SN. Strategies for reducing medication errors in the emergency department. Open Access Emergency Medicine. 2014;**6**:45-55. DOI: 10.2147/OAEM.S64174

[79] Stang AS, Wingert AS, Hartling L, Plint AC. Adverse events related to emergency department care: A systematic review. PLoS One. 2013;**8**(9):e74214. DOI: 10.1371/journal.pone.0074214

[80] Patanwala AE, Warholak TL, Sanders AB, Erstad BL. A prospective observational study of medication errors in a tertiary care emergency department. Annals of Emergency Medicine. 2010;**55**(6):522-526. DOI: 10.1016/j.annemergmed.2009.12.017

[81] Poornima P, Reshma P, Trichur Venkatakrishnan R, Rani N, Shree R, et al. Medication reconciliation and medication error prevention in an emergency department of a tertiary care hospital. Journal of Young Pharmacists. 2015;**7**(3):241-249

[82] Alsulami Z, Conroy S, Choonara I. Medication errors in the Middle East countries: A systematic review of the literature. Europian Journal of Clinical Pharmacology. 2013;**69**(4):995-1008. DOI: 10.1007/s00228-012-1435-y

[83] Thomas B, Paudyal V, MacLure K, Pallivalapila A, McLay J, El Kassem W, et al. Medication errors in hospitals in the Middle East: A systematic review of prevalence, nature, severity and contributory factors. European Journal of clinical Pharmacology. 2019;**75**(9):1269-1282. DOI: 10.1007/s00228-019-02689-y

[84] Barton L, Futtermenger J, Gaddi Y, et al. Simple prescribing errors and allergy documentation in medical hospital admissions in Australia and New Zealand. Clinical Medicine. 2012;**12**(2):119-123. DOI: 10.7861/clinmedicine.12-2-119

[85] Coombes ID, Reid C, McDougall D, et al. Pilot of a National Inpatient Medication Chart in Australia: Improving prescribing safety and enabling prescribing training. British Journal of Clinical Pharmacology. 2011;**72**(2):338-349. DOI: 10.1111/j.1365-2125.2011.03967.x

[86] Westbrook J, Lo C, Reckmann M, et al. The effectiveness of an electronic medication management system to reduce prescribing errors in hospital. HIC 18th Annual Health Informatics Conference: Informing the Business of Healthcare. 2010;**18**:96-100. DOI: 10.3316/informit.430012692310760

[87] Westbrook JI, Reckmann M, Li L, et al. Effects of two commercial electronic prescribing systems on prescribing error rates in hospital in-patients: A before and after study. PLoS Medicine. 2012;**9**(1):e1001164. DOI: 10.1371/journal.pmed.1001164

[88] Roughead EE, Semple SJ. Medication safety in acute care in Australia: Where are we now? Part 1: A review of the extent and causes of medication problems 2002-2008. Australian & New Zealand Health Policy. 2009;**6**:18. DOI: 10.1186/1743-8462-6-18

[89] Westbrook J, Woods A, Rob M, et al. Association of interruptions with an increased risk and severity of medication administration errors. Archives of Internal Medicine. 2010;**170**(8):683-690. DOI: 10.1001/archinternmed.2010.65

[90] Westbrook JI, Rob MI, Woods A, Parry D. Errors in the administration of intravenous medications in hospital and the role of correct procedures and nurse experience. BMJ Quality and Safety. 2011;**20**(12):1027-1034. DOI: 10.1136/bmjqs-2011-000089

[91] Self-care. Available from: https://www.who.int/health-topics/self-care#tab=tab

[92] What is self-care? Available from: https://www.selfcarefederation.org/what-is-self-care

[93] Yoav BS, Diana K. A life course approach to chronic disease epidemiology: Conceptual models, empirical challenges and interdisciplinary perspectives. International Journal of Epidemiology. 2002;**31**(2):285-293

[94] Julie B, Chris W, Janice S, Andy T, Jenny H. Self-management approaches for people with chronic conditions,

A review. Patient Education and Counseling. 2002;**48**(2):177-187

[95] The Epposi Barometer. Consumer perceptions of self care in Europe. In: Quantitative Study 2013. Brussels: Epposi; 2014

[96] Pollack AH, Backonja U, Miller AD, Mishra SR, Khelifi M, Kendall L, et al. Closing the gap: Supporting patients transition to self-management after hospitalization. CHI '16: Proceedings of the 2016 Conference on Human Factors in Computing Systems. 2016:5324-5336. DOI: 10.1145/2858036.2858240

[97] Self-care in Europe: Economic on Social Impact on Individuals and Society. Available from: https://aesgp.eu/resources/the-social-and-economic-value-of-self-care-aesgp-2021

Chapter 4

Microbial and Parasitic Infections in Tertiary Care: Diagnosis, Treatment, and Prevention Strategies

Adekunle Olowe, Olawumi Otutu and Rita Ayanbolade Olowe

Abstract

Microbial and parasitic infections are a significant concern in tertiary care, particularly for patients with compromised immune systems or other underlying medical conditions. In this chapter, we will focus on the diagnosis, treatment, and prevention strategies for microbial and parasitic infections in tertiary care. We will examine the different types of infections that can occur, including bacterial, viral, fungal, and parasitic infections, and the challenges associated with their diagnosis and treatment. We will also discuss the role of antimicrobial stewardship in tertiary care and the importance of appropriate use of antibiotics to prevent the development of antimicrobial resistance. Additionally, we will explore the various prevention strategies, such as vaccination, hand hygiene, and environmental disinfection, that can be used to reduce the risk of infections in tertiary care settings. Overall, this chapter highlights the importance of a proactive approach to managing microbial and parasitic infections in tertiary care, including prompt diagnosis, appropriate treatment, and effective prevention strategies.

Keywords: tertiary care, microbial infections, antimicrobial stewardship, multidisciplinary team, patient-centered care

1. Introduction

Because of the development of improved medical techniques, sophisticated diagnostic technologies, and a varied spectrum of therapeutic alternatives, the healthcare business has experienced tremendous upheaval. Notably, tertiary care, which represents the pinnacle of healthcare service and typically includes sophisticated and skilled procedures, has seen notable advancements. Providing advanced care services is fraught with problems, with microbial and parasite illnesses, especially prevalent.

These infections may represent substantial issues in the setting of tertiary care centres. Nosocomial infections endanger patients with pre-existing medical disorders and increase healthcare costs due to prolonged hospitalisation and further medical procedures. Individuals with impaired immune systems or pre-existing medical disorders are more vulnerable. In the case of these people, a minor illness can escalate into a significant medical emergency quickly.

The collection of microbial and parasitic illnesses in tertiary care settings is diverse. The pathogenic microorganisms described above, notably bacteria, viruses, fungi, and parasites, comprise a diverse group of pathogenic agents. Each cohort has unique challenges in detection, management, and mitigation. Bacterial infections have a wide range of severity, from minor to life-threatening. Likewise, viral infections may present as acute, chronic, or dormant diseases. Fungal infections often demonstrate opportunistic behaviour by preying on a weakened immune system, while parasitic infections are usually associated with specific geographic regions and environmental conditions.

Nonetheless, the complexities of these illnesses go beyond their biological variety. Identifying these situations is usually tricky owing to overlapping clinical signs, the need for specialist diagnostic equipment, and the time required to get exact results. The therapeutic domain is similarly complex. Despite the availability of several antimicrobial medications, their use must be handled with caution to prevent the development of antimicrobial resistance, which is becoming an increasingly important problem globally.

This chapter aims to provide a thorough understanding of microbiological and parasitic illnesses in tertiary healthcare. The current research intends to explore numerous illnesses, focusing on their unique characteristics and difficulties. This study aims to investigate the complexity involved in diagnosing such illnesses, as well as the fundamental principles that govern their management. It emphasises the need for antimicrobial stewardship in the current environment of rising antibiotic resistance.

In addition, the chapter will underline the need for preventative actions. In the area of infection control, it is commonly known that prevention is more effective than therapy. Vaccination, hand hygiene, ambient disinfection, and personal protective equipment are all efficient ways to reduce the risk of infection in tertiary care settings.

The fundamental goal of this chapter is to underline the critical need for a multidisciplinary, patient-centred, and proactive approach to parasite and microbial infection treatment in tertiary care settings. By proactively addressing the obstacles presented by these illnesses, such as quick diagnosis, appropriate treatment, and effective prevention, it is feasible to significantly improve patient outcomes, save healthcare costs, and, ultimately, save human lives.

2. Types of microbial and parasitic infections

In tertiary care, the variety of disease-causing bacteria and parasites is considerable. The previously described microorganisms, including bacteria, viruses, fungi, and parasites, provide unique identification, management, and prevention challenges. Bacterial infections are a significant source of worry since they may range from minor diseases to severe and possibly deadly illnesses [1]. Viral infections, such as those caused by influenza, RSV, and SARS-CoV-2, may manifest in acute, chronic, or latent forms, offering treatment issues [2]. *Candida* and *Aspergillus* are typical fungal infections, usually opportunistic and typically seen in people with impaired immune systems [3]. Despite being uncommon in developed nations, parasitic diseases remain a cause of concern for those who have gone to or are now living in locations where such illnesses are common. The causal agents of such illnesses are often identified as Cryptosporidium, Giardia, and certain helminths [4]. Understanding the many types of infections is the foundation for effective infection detection, treatment, and prevention in tertiary care.

2.1 Bacterial infections

The potential severity and breadth of clinical problems induced by bacterial infections remain significant concerns in tertiary care settings. Bacteria are responsible for various clinical symptoms, including but not limited to pneumonia, sepsis, skin, surgical wounds, and urinary tract infections [5]. Pneumonia, which is usually caused by bacterial agents such as *Streptococcus pneumoniae*, *Klebsiella pneumoniae*, and *Pseudomonas aeruginosa*, is a common disease among hospitalised patients, especially those on mechanical ventilation [6]. Bacterial pneumonia may cause severe morbidity and death, especially in those with impaired immune systems or pre-existing lung diseases. As a result, prompt detection and management are critical in improving patients' prognoses.

Bacteremia and sepsis are frequent bacterial diseases seen in tertiary care settings, generally due to the spread of a localised infection. According to Seymour et al. [7], the aetiology of these disorders is commonly related to pathogens such as *Staphylococcus aureus*, which includes methicillin-resistant *S. aureus* (MRSA) and different Enterobacteriaceae species. Infections' rapid development and high death rates demand prompt diagnosis and urgent treatment.

Bacterial infections, such as surgical site infections and skin and soft tissue infections, are common in tertiary care settings. Such infections, such as surgical lacerations or injuries, are frequently associated with integumentary system violations. They can be caused by various bacteria, including *S. aureus*, Streptococcus pyogenes, and several gram-negative bacteria [8]. The infections indicated above have the potential to cause significant consequences such as poor wound healing, abscess development, and, in severe cases, necrotizing fasciitis.

Urinary tract infections (UTIs) are a typical kind of bacterial infection in tertiary care, with *Escherichia coli*, *K. pneumoniae*, and *Proteus mirabilis* being the most common pathogens [9]. Although urinary tract infections (UTIs) are often considered minor, they may cause significant consequences in hospitalised patients, such as pyelonephritis and sepsis.

Healthcare-associated infections (HAIs), also known as nosocomial infections, are bacterial infections often observed in tertiary care settings. Nosocomial infections occur inside a healthcare institution and are caused by various bacterial pathogens. According to Weiner-Lastinger et al. [10], the presence of infections such as ventilator-associated pneumonia (VAP), catheter-associated urinary tract infections (CAUTIs), and central line-associated bloodstream infections (CLABSIs) presents significant challenges due to their potential severity and increased susceptibility to antimicrobial resistance.

Identification of bacterial infections needs a thorough examination of clinical symptoms and diagnostic methods performed in a laboratory environment. Microbiological cultures of various physiological fluids, such as blood, sputum, urine, and wound swabs, may be used in diagnostic investigations. Furthermore, molecular diagnostic methods like polymerase chain reaction (PCR) testing may be used. The rapid and exact identification of the etiological agent is critical in guiding antibiotic treatment.

Bacterial infections are frequently treated in tertiary care settings by administering systemic antibiotics. The proper antibiotic is chosen based on the discovered or suspected etiological agent's susceptibility to antibiotics, the patient's overall health, and the probability of medication interactions. In severe infections, beginning empirical broad-spectrum antibiotic treatment is routine before microbiological data are available. Following identifying the causal bacterium and its antibiotic susceptibilities, the treatment may be de-escalated, according to Barlam et al. [11].

Antimicrobial resistance is becoming more concerning, particularly in tertiary care settings where potent and broad-spectrum medicines are often used. Antibiotic abuse and usage have been linked to the rise of multidrug-resistant organisms (MDROs) such as MRSA, vancomycin-resistant enterococci (VRE), and carbapenem-resistant Enterobacteriaceae (CRE) [12]. Infections generated by Multidrug-Resistant Organisms (MDROs) may provide considerable treatment hurdles, possibly leading to poor patient outcomes.

2.2 Viral infections

The fast spread of viral infections, as well as the associated morbidity and death, are significant concerns in tertiary care settings. In these circumstances, the range of viral infections reported includes respiratory viruses such as influenza and respiratory syncytial virus (RSV), gastroenteric viruses such as Norovirus, and bloodborne viruses such as hepatitis B and C, as well as HIV [13].

In tertiary care settings, the transmission of respiratory viral infections is a substantial concern, especially in highly crowded hospital wards or during times of seasonal frequency. On a worldwide scale, influenza is a significant contributor to severe respiratory disease, with the potential to cause serious consequences such as respiratory failure, pneumonia, and death. According to Iuliano et al. [14], this is especially true for high-risk groups such as the elderly, immunocompromised persons, and those with chronic medical issues. Although RSV is usually associated with moderate sickness in children, it may cause severe disease in immunocompromised adults or have pre-existing lung disorders [15].

The advent of novel coronavirus strains, such as SARS-CoV-2, which caused the COVID-19 pandemic, has drawn attention to the potential dangers of viral infections in hospital settings in recent years. According to Huang et al. [16], the COVID-19 pandemic has had a significant impact on the tertiary healthcare sector owing to its rapid transmission, the range of illness severity ranging from mild symptoms to severe pneumonia and multi-organ failure, and the strain it has placed on healthcare resources.

Gastroenteric viruses, such as Norovirus, significantly cause morbidity in tertiary care settings. According to Lopman et al. [17], Norovirus is a leading cause of acute gastroenteritis and has been related to outbreaks in healthcare institutions due to its high infectivity and environmental durability.

Bloodborne viruses such as hepatitis B and C, as well as HIV, are also common in tertiary care settings. These diseases may be transmitted by contact with contaminated body fluids, typically due to unsafe injection practices or other breaches in infection control methods. According to Stanaway et al. [18], the presence of these viruses in the body might lead to serious health consequences such as liver disease and AIDS.

Identifying viral infections in tertiary care settings is often accomplished via molecular diagnostic methods such as polymerase chain reaction (PCR). This approach allows for the rapid and accurate identification of viral nucleic acids in patient specimens. According to Schuller et al. [19], serological testing for specific viruses may be used, in which antibodies against the virus are detected in the patient's blood.

Given the lack of specific antiviral medicines for all viral strains, managing viral infections in tertiary healthcare settings may be challenging. When antiviral therapy is available, it has the potential to significantly reduce both the frequency of illness and the number of fatalities caused by it. Antiviral medication has been shown to reduce the intensity and duration of influenza infection, especially when taken early [20]. Supportive care, such as oxygen therapy or mechanical ventilation in situations of severe respiratory viruses, is seen as a critical component of treatment.

Antiviral drugs have been more widely available in recent years, covering a more extensive range of viral illnesses. For example, the administration of direct-acting antivirals has been found to achieve cure rates surpassing 90% for hepatitis C, therefore revolutionising the treatment of this hitherto difficult-to-manage illness. The use of antiretroviral medication in the treatment of HIV has dramatically changed the care of people infected with this virus, transforming a once fatal sickness into a manageable, chronic condition [21].

Avoiding viral infections in tertiary care cannot be emphasised, especially given the limited treatment options for many viral disorders. These precautions include general infection prevention tactics, such as vaccination and hand cleanliness, and specific precautions for specific viruses. For respiratory viruses, respiratory and contact precautions are required, while standard measures are advocated for bloodborne viruses [22].

2.3 Fungal infections

Fungal infections are becoming more common in tertiary care settings, particularly among patients with impaired immune systems and those who use invasive medical equipment. Fungal pathogens, such as *Candida*, *Aspergillus*, and *Cryptococcus*, are responsible for severe infections that cause significant morbidity and death [23].

Candida species are the most common cause of fungal infections in hospitals. Candida species may cause various illnesses, from superficial mucocutaneous infections to more invasive severe disorders, including candidemia and disseminated candidiasis. Candida is a primary etiological agent of bloodstream infections connected with healthcare institutions [24], and it can potentially cause sepsis and multi-organ failure. According to Forsberg et al. [25], the introduction of Candida auris is a reason for worry because of its antibiotic resistance, ability to cause severe disease, and high fatality rates.

Aspergillus is a notable fungal infection often found in tertiary care settings. *Aspergillus* typically causes pulmonary infections, which may range from the creation of an aspergilloma, a fungal aggregation in the lungs, to the development of invasive pulmonary aspergillosis. This severe condition can spread to other internal organs. According to Patterson et al. [26], the frequency of *Aspergillus* infections is exceptionally high in people with impaired immune systems, such as those with leukaemia or who have had stem cell or organ transplantation.

Cryptococcus is a well-known fungal infection that may cause meningitis. This yeast is persistent in people living with HIV/AIDS. Despite substantial advances in antiretroviral treatment, cryptococcal meningitis remains a leading cause of death among these people [27].

The identification of fungal infections in tertiary care settings might need to be revised. Traditional approaches, like culture and microscopy, may need to be faster and more sensitive. Recent advances in diagnostic procedures, such as antigen and molecular assays, have increased efficiency and accuracy in identifying fungal infections [28].

Antifungal drugs such as azoles, echinocandins, and polyenes are extensively used to treat fungal infections. The increasing prevalence of drug-resistant fungus, such as Candida auris, provides significant challenges for medical management [29]. Furthermore, as observed by Ashbee et al. [30], administering antifungal medication may provide issues owing to possible drug-drug interactions and adverse responses, particularly in persons with numerous comorbidities or undertaking other complex regimens.

In tertiary care, fungal infections are prevented through a mix of standard infection control measures, including hand hygiene and environmental cleaning, as well as particular interventions for high-risk patients. According to Tortorano et al. [31], these approaches may include preventive antifungal medication for select immunocompromised individuals.

2.4 Parasitic infections

The incidence of parasite diseases is a significant concern in tertiary care hospitals, particularly among patients with impaired immune systems or who have visited or relocated from locations where such illnesses are common. According to Torgerson et al. [32], parasites such as Plasmodium (the agent responsible for malaria), Toxoplasma, and several forms of helminths (worms) may cause severe sickness in individuals.

Malaria caused by Plasmodium species remains a major global health issue, with an annual report of hundreds of millions of cases and hundreds of thousands of deaths, mainly in Sub-Saharan Africa [33]. Malaria is common in people who have travelled from endemic areas to tertiary care settings. According to White et al. [34], the sickness may cause symptoms ranging from mild influenza-like symptoms to serious consequences such as cerebral malaria, severe anaemia, and multi-organ failure.

The parasite Toxoplasma gondii is responsible for Toxoplasmosis, a severe illness. Although most infections cause no or relatively moderate symptoms, those with impaired immune systems, such as those with HIV/AIDS or on immunosuppressive medication, are more likely to develop serious diseases. Toxoplasmosis may cause encephalitis, a severe brain infection, and damage to other organs in patients [35].

Helminthic infections caused by several worm species may be a significant issue in tertiary care settings. The parasitic organisms described above include soil-transmitted helminths such as hookworms, roundworms, and whipworms, as well as other helminths such as schistosomes and filarial worms. Although many helminth infections cause subtle symptoms, they can potentially cause catastrophic illnesses such as malnutrition, organ dysfunction, and severe systemic disease [36].

Identifying parasite infections may be difficult, needing specific laboratory methods such as microscopy, antigen testing, or molecular studies. Suboptimal patient outcomes may occur from diagnostic delays or mistakes [37]. Antiparasitic medicines are routinely used as part of the ordinary course of therapy for parasitic illnesses. However, the particular treatment plan may vary significantly based on several circumstances, including the kind of parasite implicated and the individual patient's features. In certain circumstances, such as helminthic infections, surgical intervention may be required [38].

Preventing parasitic infections in tertiary care settings necessitates a multifaceted approach that includes universal infection control measures, such as meticulous hand hygiene and tailored interventions based on the specific parasite in question. According to Leder et al. [39], malaria prevention in travellers includes antimalarial treatment and mosquito-bite avoidance techniques.

3. Diagnosis and treatment of infections

The diagnostic and treatment procedures are critical in managing microbial and parasite illnesses in a tertiary care context. This part delves into the nuances of identifying these illnesses, the problems experienced throughout the process, the need for a timely and correct diagnosis, and the many therapy options for different infections. Furthermore, it emphasises the critical need for antibiotic stewardship, focusing on their role in a treatment strategy. To properly navigate this complex terrain, each component must be deconstructed, providing a complete understanding of the purpose and value of diagnosis and therapy in the battle against microbial and parasitic illnesses.

3.1 Challenges associated with diagnosis

Identifying and classifying microbial and parasite diseases in tertiary care settings presents several challenges. A significant worry is the wide variety of possible infections and the wide range of symptoms they might cause, which often resemble other illnesses. This characteristic may make it difficult to differentiate between infections and non-infectious diseases.

Several standard diagnostic tests, including culture and microscopy, need to be improved in terms of sensitivity, specificity, and time-consuming. The existence of these limits may result in a delay in the detection and care of medical issues, which may have negative repercussions for the patient.

According to Opota et al. [40], identifying some infections, notably certain bacteria and fungi, may be challenging owing to their complex cultivating procedure. For example, some fastidious bacteria need exact environmental parameters for multiplication, and certain varieties of fungus may take a long period to mature.

Infectious illnesses, both developing and re-emerging, are a significant source of worry. Emerging viruses, such as the SARS-CoV-2 virus that causes COVID-19, may provide problems to present diagnostic procedures, necessitating the development of innovative diagnostic tools [41].

3.2 Importance of timely and accurate diagnosis

For various reasons, accurate and timely detection of microbial and parasite diseases is critical. The timely beginning of proper therapy can reduce the severity of the disease, reduce the risk of complications, and improve patient outcomes.

A correct diagnosis helps prevent unnecessary or inappropriate treatment, such as using antibiotics for viral infections, which can contribute to antibiotic resistance [42]. Furthermore, it can potentially reduce the unnecessary use of healthcare resources.

Making an accurate diagnosis is critical in infection management and prevention. According to Siegel et al. [22], appropriate isolation and disinfection methods are critical to reducing infection inside healthcare institutions.

3.3 Treatment options for different types of infections

The treatment of microbial and parasitic diseases in tertiary care settings depends on the type of illness and the patient's unique clinical presentation. Antibiotics are the mainstay of treatment for bacterial illnesses. The type of bacterium, the location of the infection, the patient's medical history, allergies and other conditions, and the prevailing antibiotic resistance patterns in the region all influence antibiotic selection.

Antiviral medications are routinely used to treat viral infections, albeit the specific drug used depends on the kind of virus involved. Antiretroviral medication is typically used to treat HIV, but direct-acting antivirals are commonly used to treat hepatitis C.

Antifungal medications such as azoles, echinocandins, and polyenes are often used to treat fungal infections, with the exact drug chosen depending on the kind of fungus and the severity of the illness [26].

Antiparasitic medications are used to treat parasitic infections, with the kind of parasite used to choose which drug to use. According to Keiser and Utzinger [38], antimalarial medications are used to treat malaria, while antihelminthic treatments are used to treat helminth infections.

3.4 Importance of appropriate use of antibiotics

The correct use of antibiotics for bacterial infections is critical in preventing antibiotic resistance formation and spread, a significant global public health concern. According to Dellit et al. [43], practical antibiotic usage comprises only using them when essential, choosing the most appropriate antibiotic, and providing it at the proper dose and time.

Antibiotic overuse may result in the establishment of resistant bacterial strains, making future infections more difficult to treat and increasing the chance of complications and fatality [44]. Furthermore, it could encourage the spread of antibiotic-resistant germs inside healthcare institutions, exacerbating the problem.

Aside from choosing the appropriate antibiotic, it is critical to reassess the need for antibiotics in light of new evidence, such as culture results. According to Dellit et al. [43], using a de-escalation strategy is a realistic way to reduce antibiotic misuse and the chance of resistance.

Antibiotic stewardship plans have grown increasingly common in tertiary care settings in recent years to improve the effectiveness of antibiotic use. This is being done to address the previously identified problem. The courses in question use a multidisciplinary approach that draws on the experience of various healthcare experts, including infectious disease specialists, pharmacists, and microbiologists. According to Baur et al. [45], there is evidence that they may improve patient outcomes, reduce antibiotic resistance, and reduce healthcare costs.

4. Antimicrobial stewardship in tertiary care

Given the rising frequency of antimicrobial resistance and the slow progress in the discovery of new medications, it is clear that our current arsenal of antimicrobial agents requires careful management. Recognising this reality has led to the developing and implementing antimicrobial stewardship programmes, particularly at tertiary healthcare facilities that regularly meet complex and life-threatening illnesses. This section aims to offer a clear description of antimicrobial stewardship, underline the need to use antibiotics responsibly, and explain the many techniques used in tertiary care settings to improve the success of these programmes.

4.1 Definition of antimicrobial stewardship

Antimicrobial stewardship refers to structured efforts to improve and assess the prudent use of antimicrobial medicines by advocating for the most appropriate antimicrobial medication regimen, dose, treatment duration, and administration method [43]. The goal is to achieve the best clinical outcomes for antimicrobial use, reduce toxicity and other adverse outcomes, reduce healthcare costs for infections, and limit the evolution of antibiotic-resistant strains [11].

4.2 Importance of appropriate use of antibiotics

The careful use of antibiotics is a critical component of antimicrobial stewardship. Given its prominence as a significant global health concern, preventing antibiotic resistance formation and spread is critical. According to Ventola [44], the overuse and misuse of antibiotics may lead to the growth of resistant bacteria, which can complicate the treatment of future infections and increase the chance of bad outcomes and death.

According to Hicks et al. [42], improper antibiotic use may result in avoidable unpleasant responses, superimposed infections, and significantly increased medical costs. As a result, ensuring prudent antibiotic use entails more than merely avoiding resistance. It is a comprehensive strategy aimed at improving patient safety and quality of treatment.

4.3 Strategies for antimicrobial stewardship in tertiary care

Antibiotic stewardship implementation in tertiary care settings is usually marked by various measures to improve antibiotic usage efficacy. According to Baur et al. [45], the treatments above include prospective measures such as audit and feedback, formulary limitation and pre-authorisation, education, recommendations and therapeutic pathways, and antimicrobial cycling.

Prospective audit and feedback comprise a thorough examination of the acceptability of antimicrobial medication after its beginning, followed by constructive comments to the physician. Prescribers must obtain authorisation before prescribing specified antimicrobial medicines due to the introduction of formulary limitations and pre-authorisation procedures.

The primary goal of education is to improve prescribers' awareness of antimicrobials and the development of resistance. Meanwhile, guidelines and therapeutic pathways provide scientifically backed recommendations for treating specific illnesses.

Antimicrobial cycling is the systematic rotation of certain antibiotic classes to minimise the selection pressure that leads to the development of resistance. Tactics are chosen based on various factors, including the incidence of resistance, accessible assets, and organisational standards.

Furthermore, using computer-based tools for prescription and decision support may help healthcare practitioners choose appropriate antimicrobial therapies while considering the patient's clinical state and regional resistance trends [46].

Quick diagnostic assays are a promising method that may speed pathogen identification and antibiotic susceptibility profiling. This, in turn, may allow for the rapid beginning of tailored therapy while reducing the need for broad-spectrum antimicrobials, hence improving treatment efficacy.

To achieve desired results, the strategies above must be integrated into a comprehensive antimicrobial stewardship programme supported by hospital leadership, involving all healthcare professionals involved in antimicrobial use and consistently monitoring and providing feedback on antimicrobial use and resistance to prescribers [11].

5. Prevention strategies

Along with diagnosis and treatment, prevention of microbial and parasite diseases is an equally important element of treating these illnesses, especially in tertiary care settings. The importance of prevention cannot be overstated in an environment where vulnerable persons are being served. Prophylactic methods are typically the primary means of protection, reducing the chance of infection and spread. This section delves into five key preventative strategies: vaccination, hand hygiene, environmental disinfection, use of personal protective equipment, and isolation measures. Implementing these measures leads to a complete and multifaceted approach to infection prevention in tertiary care settings.

5.1 Vaccination

Immunisation is a critical component in protecting against infectious illnesses. Vaccines protect against prospective diseases by inducing the body's immune response to particular microorganisms. The Centres for Disease Control and Prevention (CDC) and the World Health Organisation (WHO) advise the delivery of numerous vaccinations to persons, especially those who are vulnerable to severe diseases, such as tertiary care patients [47, 48].

Aside from protecting the vaccinated person, achieving high vaccination coverage within a community may result in herd immunity, lowering the overall frequency of the disease and protecting unvaccinated people [49]. Healthcare worker vaccination is critical in controlling healthcare-associated illnesses, reducing the possibility of transmission to patients [50].

5.2 Hand hygiene

Hand hygiene is a very effective strategy for reducing illness transmission inside healthcare settings. The procedure comprises systematically and thoroughly cleaning hands with soap and water or an alcohol-based hand sanitiser. The World Health Organisation has produced a set of recommendations known as the "5 Moments for Hand Hygiene," which define when healthcare professionals should practise hand hygiene. These include times before and after contact with a patient, before and after a clean/aseptic operation, after exposure to body fluids, and after interaction with the patient's surroundings [51].

5.3 Environmental disinfection

Given the enormous influence of the environment in this respect, environmental disinfection is critical in reducing the spread of several healthcare-associated diseases. As a result, it is an essential part of infection prevention in tertiary care settings. According to Carling [52], the suggested course of action is periodic cleaning and sanitization of numerous surfaces and things that have the potential to harbour hazardous germs, such as bed rails, bedside tables, medical equipment, and bathroom fixtures.

Disinfection of the environment may be accomplished using a variety of goods and technologies, including detergents, chemical disinfectants, and sophisticated approaches such as ultraviolet radiation or hydrogen peroxide vapour. The approach used is determined by several criteria, including the nature of the surface or item, the kind of pathogen, and the healthcare setting [53].

5.4 Personal Protective Equipment (PPE)

Personal Protective Equipment (PPE) such as gloves, gowns, masks, and eye protection are critical in protecting healthcare personnel from infectious pathogens. Furthermore, as Siegel et al. [22] point out, PPE is a preventative strategy against disease transmission from healthcare personnel to patients or from one patient to another. Combining Personal Protective Equipment (PPE) with other measures, such as hand cleanliness, is suggested for successful infection prevention.

5.5 Isolation precautions

Isolation measures are a preventative technique to prevent pathogen transmission from infected or colonised patients to other patients, healthcare personnel, or visitors. Standard precautions and transmission-based precautions are the two kinds of precautions advised for limiting the spread of illnesses in healthcare settings. Transmission-based precautions, such as contact, droplet, and airborne precautions, should be implemented for patients who are either confirmed or suspected to be infected or colonised with specific pathogens that can be transmitted through direct contact, large respiratory droplets, or tiny airborne droplets [22].

These preventative measures' efficiency depends on healthcare staff receiving constant training and instruction, adhering to specified criteria, conducting frequent audits, and providing feedback. Furthermore, these procedures must be tailored to different tertiary care centres' specific needs and conditions. This requires considering characteristics such as patient demographics, service offerings, and infection rates in the area. Implementing and maintaining preventative techniques in tertiary care settings may result in a significant decrease in the risk of microbial and parasite infections, an improvement in patient outcomes, and an increase in overall care quality.

6. Conclusion

The current chapter has looked at the numerous categories of microbial and parasite diseases in tertiary care settings, the difficulties involved in their diagnosis, treatment options, and the need for prevention. The importance of precise and prompt diagnosis has been emphasised focusing on providing detailed insights into the pathogen's identity and susceptibility to antimicrobial agents. The chapter also examined several therapy options, recognising the importance of judicious antibiotic dosing and antimicrobial stewardship in tackling the global threat of antimicrobial resistance.

Infection management involves applying basic preventative techniques such as immunisation, hand hygiene, environmental disinfection, personal protective equipment, and isolation procedures. Combining several treatments may result in a holistic strategy that reduces infection risk in tertiary care settings.

Prospective innovations in this subject are expected to progress due to technical breakthroughs, changes in infection epidemiology, and the ongoing problem of antibiotic resistance, both in research and practical applications. Future studies should prioritise the development of innovative diagnostic tools and medicines, identify practical ways for antimicrobial stewardship and infection prevention, and evaluate their impact on patient outcomes and healthcare expenses. It is critical to research innovative approaches, such as machine learning and predictive modelling, to improve infection detection and control.

Continuous education and training of healthcare staff, the adoption of evidence-based standards and procedures, and a patient-centric approach that addresses each patient's particular needs and preferences are all required for the practical implementation of healthcare. Furthermore, it is critical to emphasise the need for a multidisciplinary approach in treating such diseases, in which doctors, chemists, microbiologists, infection preventionists, and other healthcare professionals work together to provide the best possible care.

In conclusion, managing microbial and parasite diseases in tertiary care settings is complex but necessary. It is possible to reduce the burden of these illnesses, improve patient outcomes, and ensure the long-term viability of our healthcare systems by adopting timely diagnosis, appropriate treatment, effective preventative measures, and a commitment to continuous improvement.

Author details

Adekunle Olowe[1*], Olawumi Otutu[1] and Rita Ayanbolade Olowe[1,2]

1 Department of Medical Microbiology and Parasitology, College of Health Sciences, Oyo, Oyo State, Nigeria

2 Research Ethics Unit, UNIOSUN Teaching Hospital, Osogbo, Osun State, Nigeria

*Address all correspondence to: oaolowe@lautech.edu.ng

References

[1] Bennett JE, Dolin R, Blaser MJ. Mandell, Douglas, and Bennett's Principles and Practice of Infectious Diseases E-book. Elsevier Health Sciences; 2019

[2] Howley PM, Knipe DM, Enquist LW. Fields Virology: Fundamentals. Lippincott Williams & Wilkins; 2023

[3] Kauffman CA. Fungal infections. Infectious Disease in the Aging: A Clinical Handbook. 2009;**2009**:347-366

[4] Garcia LS, Procop GW. Diagnostic Medical Parasitology: Manual of Commercial Methods in Clinical Microbiology. International Edition; 2016. pp. 284-308

[5] Magill SS, Edwards JR, Bamberg W, Beldavs ZG, Dumyati G, Kainer MA, et al. Multistate point-prevalence survey of health care–associated infections. New England Journal of Medicine. 2014;**370**(13):1198-1208

[6] Kalil AC, Metersky ML, Klompas M, Muscedere J, Sweeney DA, Palmer LB, et al. Management of adults with hospital-acquired and ventilator-associated pneumonia: 2016 clinical practice guidelines by the Infectious Diseases Society of America and the American Thoracic Society. Clinical Infectious Diseases. 2016;**63**(5):e61-e111

[7] Seymour CW, Liu VX, Iwashyna TJ, Brunkhorst FM, Rea TD, Scherag A, et al. Assessment of clinical criteria for sepsis: For the third international consensus definitions for Sepsis and septic shock (Sepsis-3). JAMA. 2016;**315**(8):762-774

[8] Anderson DJ, Podgorny K, Berríos-Torres SI, Bratzler DW, Dellinger EP, Greene L, et al. Strategies to prevent surgical site infections in acute care hospitals: 2014 update. Infection Control & Hospital Epidemiology. 2014;**35**(S2):S66-S88

[9] Foxman B. Urinary tract infection syndromes: Occurrence, recurrence, bacteriology, risk factors, and disease burden. Infectious Disease Clinics. 2014;**28**(1):1-13

[10] Weiner-Lastinger LM, Abner S, Edwards JR, Kallen AJ, Karlsson M, Magill SS, et al. Antimicrobial-resistant pathogens associated with adult healthcare-associated infections: Summary of data reported to the National Healthcare Safety Network, 2015-2017. Infection Control & Hospital Epidemiology. 2020;**41**(1):1-18

[11] Barlam TF, Cosgrove SE, Abbo LM, MacDougall C, Schuetz AN, Septimus EJ, et al. Implementing an antibiotic stewardship program: Guidelines by the Infectious Diseases Society of America and the Society for Healthcare Epidemiology of America. Clinical Infectious Diseases. 2016;**62**(10):e51-e77

[12] Centers for Disease Control and Prevention. Antibiotic Resistance Threats in the United States, 2019. Atlanta, GA: US Department of Health and Human Services, CDC; 2019

[13] Hibberd PL, Rubin RH. Clinical aspects of fungal infection in organ transplant recipients. Clinical Infectious Diseases. 1994;**19**(Supplement_1):S33-S40

[14] Iuliano AD, Roguski KM, Chang HH, Muscatello DJ, Palekar R, Tempia S, et al. Estimates of global

seasonal influenza-associated respiratory mortality: A modelling study. The Lancet. 2018;**391**(10127):1285-1300

[15] Falsey AR, Hennessey PA, Formica MA, Cox C, Walsh EE. Respiratory syncytial virus infection in elderly and high-risk adults. New England Journal of Medicine. 2005;**352**(17):1749-1759

[16] Huang C, Wang Y, Li X, Ren L, Zhao J, Hu Y, et al. Clinical features of patients infected with 2019 novel coronavirus in Wuhan, China. The Lancet. 2020;**395**(10223):497-506

[17] Lopman BA, Steele D, Kirkwood CD, Parashar UD. The vast and varied global burden of norovirus: Prospects for prevention and control. PLoS Medicine. 2016;**13**(4):e1001999

[18] Stanaway JD, Flaxman AD, Naghavi M, Fitzmaurice C, Vos T, Abubakar I, et al. The global burden of viral hepatitis from 1990 to 2013: Findings from the global burden of disease study 2013. The Lancet. 2016;**388**(10049):1081-1088

[19] Schuller M, Sloots TP, James GS, Halliday CL, Carter IW. PCR for clinical microbiology. An Australian and International Perspective. 2010;**2010**:191193

[20] Uyeki TM, Bernstein HH, Bradley JS, Englund JA, File TM Jr, Fry AM, et al. Clinical practice guidelines by the Infectious Diseases Society of America: 2018 update on diagnosis, treatment, chemoprophylaxis, and institutional outbreak management of seasonal influenza. Clinical Infectious Diseases. 2019;**68**(6):e1-e47

[21] Deeks SG, Lewin SR, Havlir DV. The end of AIDS: HIV infection as a chronic disease. The Lancet. 2013;**382**(9903):1525-1533

[22] Siegel JD, Rhinehart E, Jackson M, Chiarello L. 2007 guideline for isolation precautions: Preventing transmission of infectious agents in health care settings. American Journal of Infection Control. 2007;**35**(10):S65-S164

[23] Brown GD, Denning DW, Gow NA, Levitz SM, Netea MG, White TC. Hidden killers: Human fungal infections. Science Translational Medicine. 2012;**4**(165):165rv13-165rv13

[24] Pappas PG, Lionakis MS, Arendrup MC, Ostrosky-Zeichner L, Kullberg BJ. Invasive candidiasis. Nature Reviews Disease Primers. 2018;**4**(1):1-20

[25] Forsberg K, Woodworth K, Walters M, Berkow EL, Jackson B, Chiller T, et al. *Candida auris*: The recent emergence of a multidrug-resistant fungal pathogen. Medical Mycology. 2019;**57**(1):1-12

[26] Patterson TF, Thompson GR III, Denning DW, Fishman JA, Hadley S, Herbrecht R, et al. Practice guidelines for the diagnosis and management of aspergillosis: 2016 update by the Infectious Diseases Society of America. Clinical Infectious Diseases. 2016;**63**(4):e1-e60

[27] Rajasingham R, Smith RM, Park BJ, Jarvis JN, Govender NP, Chiller TM, et al. Global burden of disease of HIV-associated cryptococcal meningitis: An updated analysis. The Lancet Infectious Diseases. 2017;**17**(8):873-881

[28] Clancy CJ, Nguyen MH. Diagnosing invasive candidiasis. Journal of Clinical Microbiology. 2018;**56**(5):e01909-e01917

[29] Lockhart SR, Etienne KA, Vallabhaneni S, Farooqi J, Chowdhary A,

GovenderNP,etal.Simultaneousemergence of multidrug-resistant Candida auris on 3 continents confirmed by whole-genome sequencing and epidemiological analyses. Clinical Infectious Diseases. 2017;**64**(2):134-140

[30] Ashbee HR, Barnes RA, Johnson EM, Richardson MD, Gorton R, Hope WW. Therapeutic drug monitoring (TDM) of antifungal agents: Guidelines from the British Society for Medical Mycology. Journal of Antimicrobial Chemotherapy. 2014;**69**(5):1162-1176

[31] Tortorano AM, Richardson M, Roilides E, Van Diepeningen A, Caira M, Munoz P, et al. ESCMID and ECMM joint guidelines on diagnosis and management of hyalohyphomycosis: Fusarium spp., Scedosporium spp. and others. Clinical Microbiology and Infection. 2014;**20**:27-46

[32] Torgerson PR, Devleesschauwer B, Praet N, Speybroeck N, Willingham AL, Kasuga F, et al. World Health Organization estimates of the global and regional disease burden of 11 foodborne parasitic diseases, 2010: A data synthesis. PLoS Medicine. 2015;**12**(12):e1001920

[33] World Health Organization. World Malaria Report 2020: 20 years of Global Progress and Challenges. World Health Organization; 2020

[34] White NJ, Pukrittayakamee S, Hien TT, Faiz MA, Mokuolu OA, Dondorp AM. Malaria. The Lancet. 2014;**383**(9918):723-735

[35] Montoya JG, Liesenfeld O. Toxoplasmosis. Lancet. 2004;**363**:1965-1976

[36] Bethony J, Brooker S, Albonico M, Geiger SM, Loukas A, Diemert D, et al. Soil-transmitted helminth infections: Ascariasis, trichuriasis, and hookworm. The Lancet. 2006;**367**(9521):1521-1532

[37] Jung BK, Chai JY. Parasitology: A conceptual approach. The Korean Journal of Parasitology. 2015;**53**(4):507

[38] Keiser J, Utzinger J. The drugs we have and the drugs we need against major helminth infections. Advances in Parasitology. 2010;**73**:197-230

[39] Leder K, Torresi J, Libman MD, Cramer JP, Castelli F, Schlagenhauf P, et al. GeoSentinel surveillance of illness in returned travelers, 2007-2011. Annals of Internal Medicine. 2013;**158**(6):456-468

[40] Opota O, Croxatto A, Prod'hom G, Greub G. Blood culture-based diagnosis of bacteraemia: State of the art. Clinical Microbiology and Infection. 2015;**21**(4):313-322

[41] Guan WJ, Ni ZY, Hu Y, Liang WH, Ou CQ, He JX, et al. Clinical characteristics of coronavirus disease 2019 in China. New England Journal of Medicine. 2020;**382**(18):1708-1720

[42] Hicks LA, Taylor TH Jr, Hunkler RJ. US outpatient antibiotic prescribing, 2010. New England Journal of Medicine. 2013;**368**(15):1461-1462

[43] Dellit TH, Owens RC, McGowan JE, Gerding DN, Weinstein RA, Burke JP, et al. Infectious Diseases Society of America and the Society for Healthcare Epidemiology of America guidelines for developing an institutional program to enhance antimicrobial stewardship. Clinical Infectious Diseases. 2007;**44**(2):159-177

[44] Ventola CL. The antibiotic resistance crisis: Part 1: Causes and threats. Pharmacy and Therapeutics. 2015;**40**(4):277

[45] Baur D, Gladstone BP, Burkert F, Carrara E, Foschi F, Döbele S, et al.

Effect of antibiotic stewardship on the incidence of infection and colonisation with antibiotic-resistant bacteria and Clostridium difficile infection: A systematic review and meta-analysis. The Lancet Infectious Diseases. 2017;**17**(9):990-1001

[46] Marston HD, Dixon DM, Knisely JM, Palmore TN, Fauci AS. Antimicrobial resistance. Jama. 2016;**316**(11):1193-1204

[47] World Health Organization (WHO). Vaccines and immunization. 2020. Retrieved from: https://www.who.int/health-topics/vaccines-and-immunization

[48] Centers for Disease Control and Prevention (CDC). Vaccines & immunizations. 2020. Retrieved from: https://www.cdc.gov/vaccines/index.html

[49] Fine P, Eames K, Heymann DL. "Herd immunity": A rough guide. Clinical Infectious Diseases. 2011;**52**(7):911-916

[50] Haviari S, Bénet T, Saadatian-Elahi M, André P, Loulergue P, Vanhems P. Vaccination of healthcare workers: A review. Human Vaccines & Immunotherapeutics. 2015;**11**(11):2522-2537

[51] World Health Organization (WHO). WHO Guidelines on Hand Hygiene in Health Care. 2009. Retrieved from: https://www.who.int/publications/i/item/9789241597906

[52] Carling PC. Optimizing health care environmental hygiene. Infectious Disease Clinics. 2016;**30**(3):639-660

[53] Boyce JM. Modern technologies for improving cleaning and disinfection of environmental surfaces in hospitals. Antimicrobial Resistance & Infection Control. 2016;**5**(1):1-10

Chapter 5

Diabetic Macular Edema, Clinicopathologic and Keys for Management

Ahmed Darwish

Abstract

Diabetic retinopathy (DR) is one of the leading causes of blindness worldwide. It usually begins several years after the onset of diabetes. In the early stages, there are relatively mild retinal changes, the most important of which, regarding visual acuity (VA) affection, is diabetic macular edema (DME). Recently, the development of optical coherence tomography (OCT) and optical coherence tomography angiography (OCTA) greatly changed the treatment strategy of this part of diabetic retinopathy, particularly with the development of more advanced laser technologies as micropulse laser and more effective and longer acting anti-VEGF and steroid intravitreal medications and the advances in pars plana vitrectomy (PPV) techniques. In this chapter, all those points will be highlighted with how to prevent the progression of retinopathy to save as much as could be saved of the visual function.

Keywords: diabetes, macular edema, OCT, anti-VEGF, laser, steroids

1. Introduction

Diabetic retinopathy (DR) is one of the most handicapping complications of diabetes, as it threatens the vision of about 5–10% of patients suffering from diabetes, many of whom are in the working age group [1–4]. In the following sections, we shall concentrate on the pathogenesis, diagnosis and management of the early visually threatening complication of diabetic retinopathy, namely diabetic macular edema (DME).

2. Early preclinical changes of diabetic retinopathy

Chronic hyperglycemia affects both the microvascular and neural components of the retina by increasing the oxidative stress, inflammation and hypoxia (**Figure 1**) [5]. As a type of metabolic autoregulation, the earliest changes that occur in the retinal microvasculature secondary to hyperglycemia are retinal blood vessel dilatation and blood flow changes. Pericyte apoptosis secondary to hyperglycemia is also an early event in this pathology, and because pericytes provide structural support to the retinal capillary walls, outpouching of the capillary walls occurs forming microaneurysms, the earliest clinical sign that can be overlooked in very early stages [6, 7]. Glial cell activation and

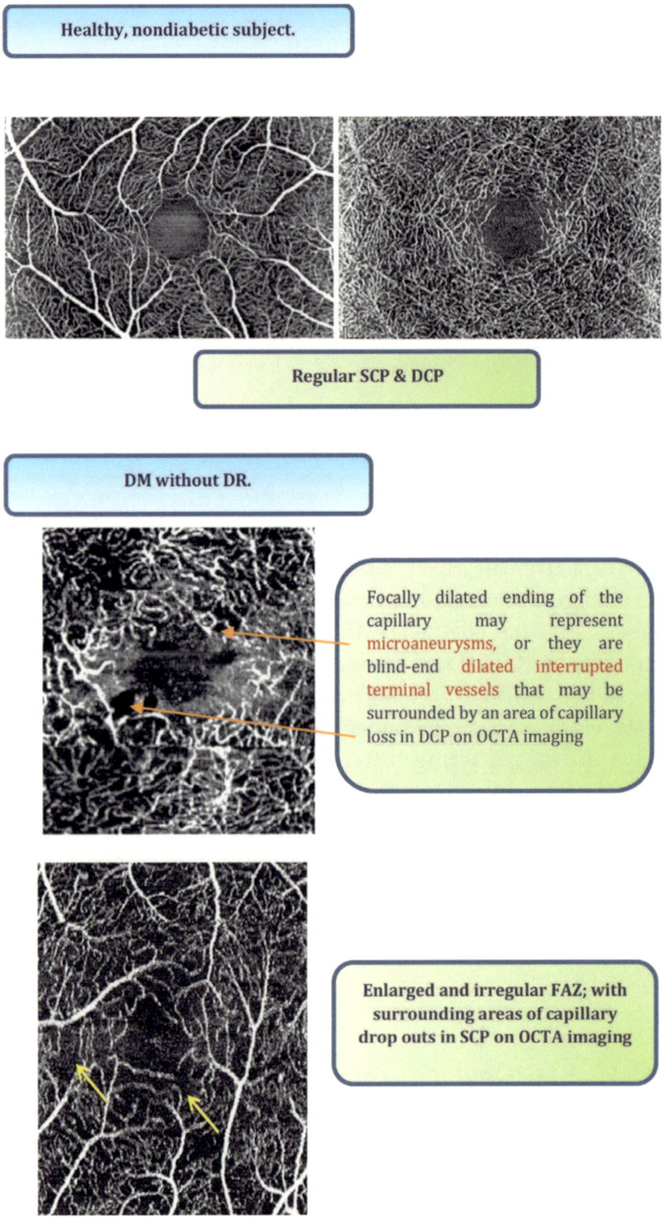

Figure 1.
Early preclinical changes of diabetic retinopathy.

neural apoptosis lead to ganglion cell death, with consequent thinning of the ganglion cell layer preclinical to the signs of diabetic retinopathy seen on fundus examination [8]. Using optical coherence tomography angiography (OCT angiography) (OCTA), the foveal avascular zone (FAZ) in both the superficial and deep capillary plexuses (SCP and DCP) was found to be larger and irregular due to perifoveal capillary loss with more tortuosity, beading and focally dilated endings of capillaries. These findings were found to be more pronounced when diabetes was associated with hypertension [8].

3. Diabetic macular edema (DME)

3.1 Pathogenesis

3.1.1 The normal blood retinal barrier (BRB) in healthy subjects

The inner and outer retinal barriers keep the retina immune privileged and regulate fluid and molecular entry and drainage into and to the outside of the retina keeping the retina in a dehydrated state [9].

The inner blood retinal barrier (retinal blood vessel walls) is formed by tight junctions (zonula occludens (ZO)) between endothelial cells, adherens junctions between pericyte cytoskeleton and endothelial cells and glial cell processes wrap around retinal capillaries [10]. Astrocytes and Müller cells stabilize the tight junctions between endothelial cells and ensheath vascular plexuses [11]. Finally, microglia produce soluble factors important for vesicular communication necessary for the maintenance of the inner blood retinal barrier [12, 13].

The outer blood retinal barrier is formed of junctional complexes between retinal pigment epithelial (RPE) cells formed of tight, adherens and gap junctions separating the neurosensory retina from the fenestrated choriocapillaris. It controls the transport of fluid and solutes into and to the outside of the retina to maintain its integrity [14, 15].

3.1.2 Pathologic alterations in diabetic macular edema

Microglia monitor the physiological microenvironment in the retina and can detect early signs of hyperglycemia leading to their activation [16]. Activation of microglial cells is usually associated with perivasculitis with consequent release of inflammatory mediators, including vascular endothelial growth factor (VEGF), tumor necrosis factor alpha (TNF-α), interleukin 6 (IL-6) and monocyte chemotactic protein-1 (MCP-1), resulting in extension of the inflammation from the inner retina to all retinal layers with breakdown of the blood retinal barrier, increased vascular permeability and retinal neuronal damage [17–20].

Hyperglycemia upregulates intercellular adhesion molecule-1 (ICAM-1) which together with vascular cell adhesion molecule mediate leukocyte adhesion to the vascular endothelium (leukostasis), resulting in vascular damage and capillary nonperfusion. Additionally, leukocytes share in microvascular damage by the release of cytokines and superoxide [21].

Inflammation and hypoxia adversely affect the functions of Müller cells, altering their potassium channels with consequent accumulation of intracellular fluids [22, 23]. Both inflammation and hypoxia also stimulate retinal Müller cells to produce VEGF, tumor necrosis factor alpha (TNF-α), interleukin 1β (IL-1β) and prostaglandins, all of which contribute to the increased vascular permeability [24, 25]. On the other hand, Müller cells aggravate inflammation through stimulation of cluster of differentiation (CD) 40 and through the release of adenosine triphosphate (ATP) which promotes microglial inflammation [26].

Vascular endothelial growth factor, a main factor in the progression of DME and proliferative diabetic retinopathy (PDR) (**Figure 2**), is upregulated through several pathways, particularly the activation of hypoxia-inducible factor 1 (HIF-1) [27]

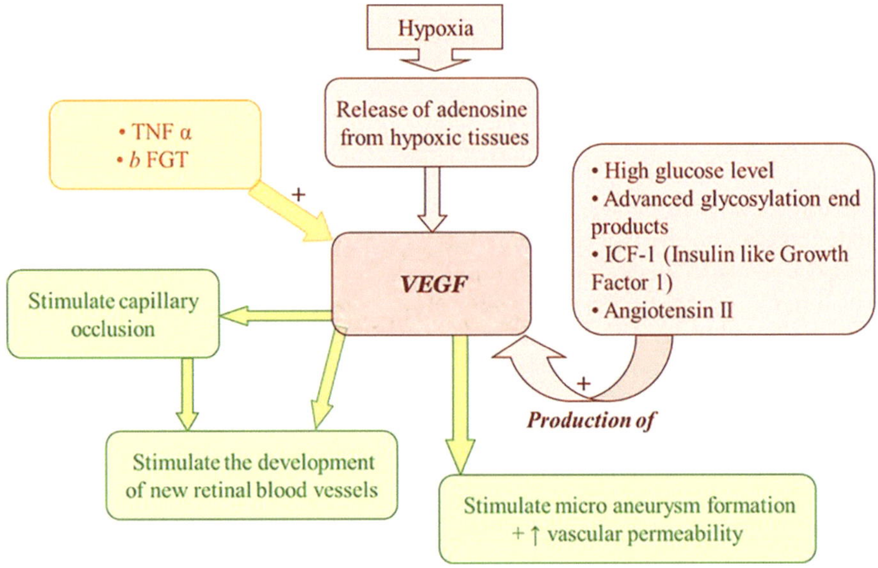

Figure 2.
VEGF in DME and PDR.

and phospholipase A2 (PLA2) [28]. VEGF both increases vascular permeability by promoting phosphorylation of tight junction proteins, such as occludin and zonula occludens-1 (ZO-1) [29], in addition to its effect in promoting angiogenesis through the activation of mitogen-activated protein (MAP) [30].

Other angiogenic factors, particularly angioprotein 2 (Ang-2), an antagonist to endothelial receptor tyrosine kinase (Tie2), has been shown to promote vascular leakage in diabetic retina (**Figure 3**) [31].

Reactive oxygen species (ROS) are an important link between hyperglycemia and the main pathways responsible for hyperglycemic damage. Although mitochondrial production is an important source of ROS [32], yet more recently it was proved that ROS derived from nicotinamide adenine dinucleotide phosphate (NADPH) oxidase is involved to a higher extent in the process of pericyte apoptosis on exposure to high glucose levels [33]. High glucose could stimulate ROS production through protein kinase C (PKC) β-dependent phosphorylation of the p47phox (the phagocyte NADPH oxidase/NOX_2 organizer) subunit (involved in the activation of NADPH oxidase) [34].

Diabetic macular edema is also associated with RPE dysfunction and impaired control of transport of water from the subretinal space into the choriocapillaris and vice versa [14].

3.2 Pretreatment evaluation of DME

3.2.1 Screening

All diabetic patients should perform baseline screening with full ophthalmological examination and imaging (fluorescein angiography (FA) together with OCT). Although FA has long been used for the diagnosis of diabetic retinopathy (DR), yet the intravenous dye injection can cause some side effects [35]. In addition, FA does

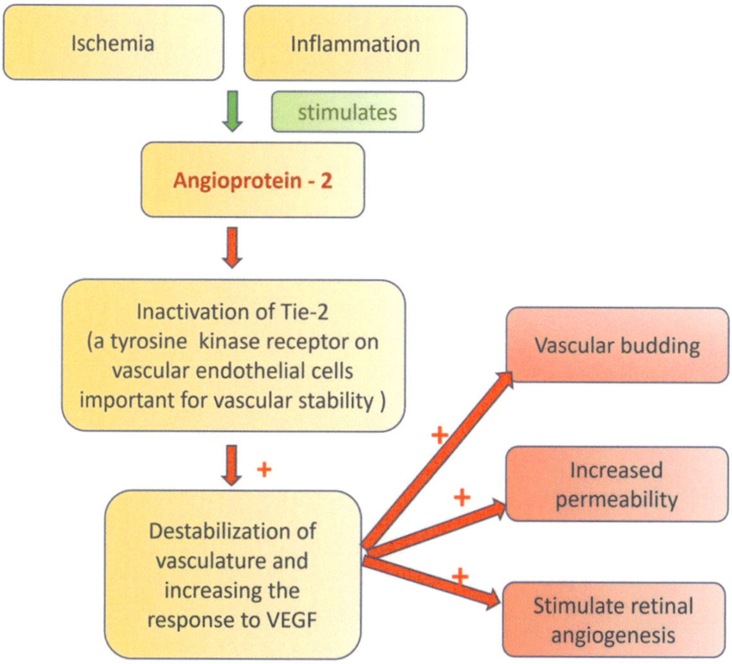

Figure 3.
Role of angioprotein-2 in increasing vascular permeability and DME.

not identify or separate the pathologies in the superficial and deep capillary networks of the retina and the leaking fluorescein dye may obscure the alterations in vascular morphology. All FA drawbacks are recently solved by the use of OCTA [36].

In type 1 diabetes mellitus (type 1 DM), it is usually advised to do the first ophthalmologic examination 5 years after the discovery of diabetes mellitus (DM), while in type 2 diabetes mellitus (type 2 DM), the examination is done once DM is diagnosed, then annually or earlier as needed [37].

3.2.2 Classifications of DME

Several attempts have been carried out to classify DME. A summary of these classifications is given as follows:

1. Center-involved vs. noncenter-involved DME [38].

2. Vasogenic vs. nonvasogenic DME: [6]

    a. The vasogenic type was defined as retinal thickening with visible retinal vascular abnormalities detectable on biomicroscopy and fundus photography (focally grouped microaneurysm and dilated capillaries) at the macular region usually associated with lipid exudates.

    b. The nonvasogenic type, on the other hand, was defined as retinal thickening with no visible vascular dilations and probably no lipid exudates detectable on biomicroscopy and fundus photography.

c. Mixed type: It is either a vasogenic or a nonvasogenic type associated with retinal thickening and detectable traction on OCT examination (**Figure 4**).

3. Optical coherence tomography (OCT) classification (conventional OCT imaging):

Three types of optical coherence tomography are recognized:

a. Diffuse thickening type (sponge-like diffuse retinal thickening) (**Figure 5**), which results from increased vascular permeability and breakdown of the inner blood retinal barrier secondary to inflammation and oxidative stress [14].

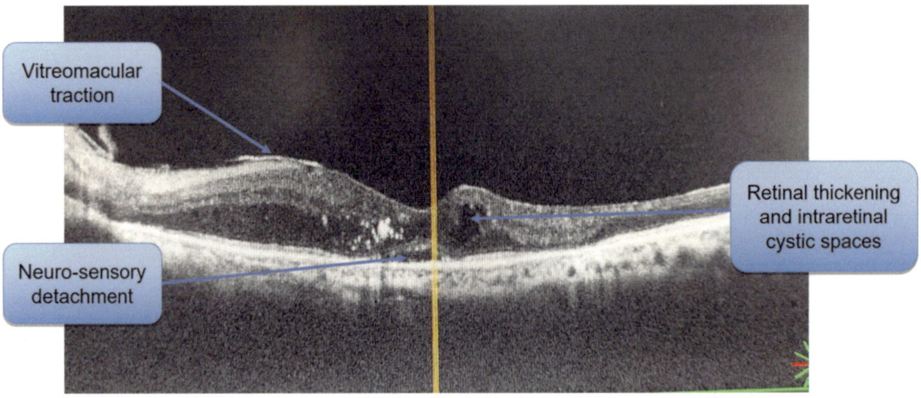

Figure 4.
Mixed type of DME.

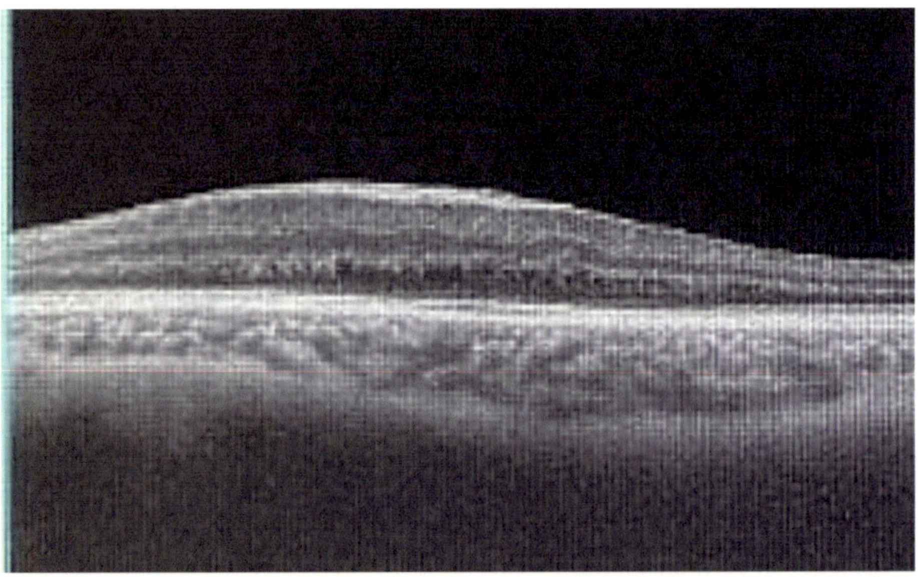

Figure 5.
Diffuse thickening type of DME.

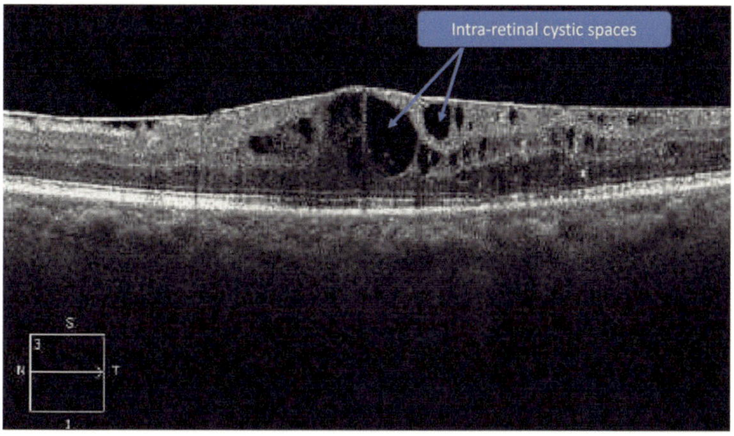

Figure 6.
Cystoid macular edema (CME) type.

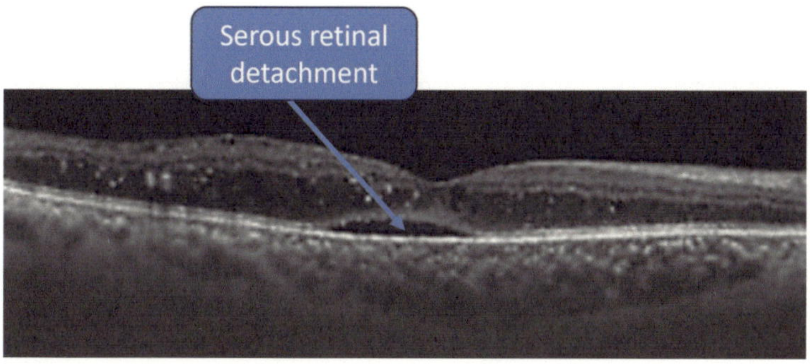

Figure 7.
Serous retinal detachment (SRD) type.

b. Cystoid macular edema (CME) type (thickening of fovea with intraretinal cystoid changes) (**Figure 6**) produced by a combination of production of prostaglandins and inflammatory cytokines together with ischemia, particularly in the deep capillary plexus around the cystoid spaces (demonstrated by OCTA) and finally necrosis of Müller cells [22].

c. Serous retinal detachment (SRD) type (thickening of fovea with subretinal fluid) (**Figure 7**): Probably, detachment begins by increased permeability of the choriocapillaris (evidenced by thickened subfoveal choroid) followed by a breakdown of the outer blood retinal barrier and damage of the external limiting membrane (ELM) secondary to inflammation (as evidenced by the elevation of interleukin 6 (IL-6) levels in this subtype [14]).

4. Spectral domain optical coherence tomography grading system of diabetic maculopathy (**Table 1**) [38].

5. En face image-based classification of diabetic macular edema using swept source optical coherence tomography: [35]

Parameter	Grade	Description
Thickening	0	Less than 10% increase above upper normal values
	1	More than 10% but less than 30% increase above upper normal values
	2	More than 30% increase above upper normal values
Cysts (round, minimally reflective spaces within the neurosensory retina)	0	Absent
	1	Mild
	2	Moderate
	3	Severe
Ellipsoid zone (EZ) and/or ELM status (the first and the second hyperreflective bands of the four outermost layers on OCT, respectively)	0	Intact
	1	Disrupted
	2	Absent
Disorganization of the inner retinal layers (DRIL) (loss of clear demarcation between the ganglion cell-inner plexiform layer complex, the inner nuclear layer and the outer plexiform layer in the central fovea)	0	Absent
	1	Present
Hyperreflective foci (1) reflectivity similar to that of nerve fiber layer; (2) absence of backshadowing; and (3) <30 μm diameter	0	Less than 30 in number
	1	More than 30 in number
Subretinal fluid (subfoveal neurosensory hyporeflective detachment due to fluid accumulation)	0	Absent
	1	Present
Vitreoretinal relationship	0	Absence of any visible adhesion or traction between vitreous cortex and retina
	1	Incomplete posterior vitreous detachment
	2	Posterior vitreous detachment
	3	Vitreomacular traction
	4	Epiretinal membrane

Table 1.
Optical coherence tomography (OCT) grading of diabetic macular edema (DME).

Segment	Layers included	Parameter
Segment 1	Comprises inner nuclear layer, outer plexiform layer including Henle's fiber layer	No fluid
		Foveal cystoid space
		Parafoveal cystoid space
		Diffuse fluid
Segment 2	Mainly comprises the outer nuclear layer	No fluid
		Diffuse fluid
		Subretinal fluid
		Diffuse fluid with subretinal fluid

Table 2.
En face image-based classification of diabetic macular edema.

The idea of this classification is to construct en face images from three-dimensional (3D) images to visualize and localize the extent of the area of fluid at a specific retinal depth in cases of DME (**Table 2**).

Conclusions drawn from this classification were as follows:

First, the presence of fluid in Segment 2 resulted in a significantly worse visual outcome as compared to cases without fluid in this area, which is probably because of the disturbed oxygenation and elimination of metabolites from the layer of photoreceptors.

Second conclusion was that the extent of fluid in Segment 1 did not affect the final visual acuity (VA) in DME [35].

3.2.3 Baseline predictors for a good treatment response based on OCT findings

Several pretreatment criteria were found to be of prognostic value as regards better vision gain posttreatment, and these predictors include; less subretinal fluid (SRF) and few intraretinal cystoid spaces (IRC) and no vitreomacular traction (VMT) (**Figure 8**) [39].

Better vision gain is also achieved if there was no disruption or disorganization of the inner retinal layers (DRIL) [40] and if there was preservation of the ellipsoid zone (EZ) and external limiting membrane (ELM) [41].

A thin subfoveal choroid at baseline may predict unfavorable posttreatment visual acuity, while eyes with a thicker baseline subfoveal choroidal thickness had better short-term anatomic and functional responses [42].

Several OCTA biomarkers have been found to be valuable in the determination of the degree of retinal ischemia and these include two FAZ biomarkers, namely foveal avascular zone area (FAZ-A) and the irregularity in the contour of the foveal avascular zone contour irregularities (FAZ-CI) and three vessel biomarkers, namely the tortuosity of retinal vessels (VT), the average vessel caliber (AVC) and the density of retinal vessels (VD) [43].

3.2.4 Pretreatment systemic monitoring

Systemic risk factors for progression of diabetic macular edema should be controlled to provide a suitable environment for ocular treatment to give better and longer lasting favorable results;

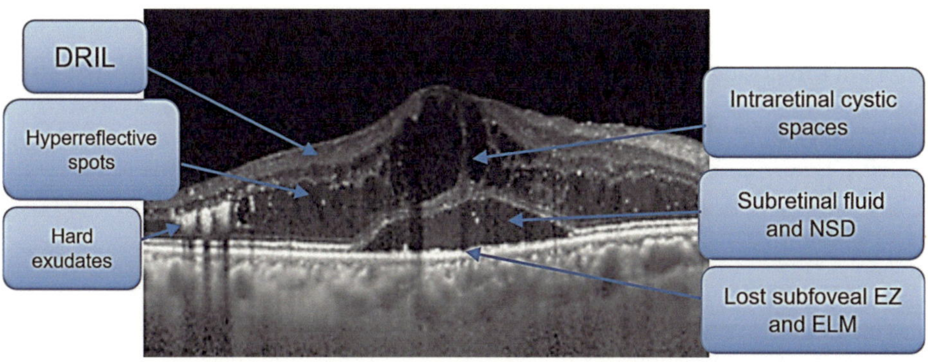

Figure 8.
Base line predictors for an unfavorable treatment response based on OCT findings.

Multiple randomized clinical trials demonstrated the benefits of both controlled blood sugar level and arterial blood pressure in the reduction of retinopathy progression [44–49]. The American Diabetes Association mentioned that the glycated hemoglobin (HbA1c) level should not exceed 7%, while the arterial blood pressure level should be kept under 130/80 mmHg and total lipids under 100 mg/dL [50], in addition, however, treatment should not be delayed to correct all systemic parameters [51–53].

Other parameters that are also to be taken into consideration are smoking cessation [54, 55], weight loss if required for a normal body mass index [55], renal impairment [54, 55] and sleep apnea [55], as all of those factors have an impact on the results of management of DME.

3.3 Treatment options

3.3.1 Laser treatment

For diabetic macular edema, laser photocoagulation was the gold standard for treatment until the introduction of anti-VEGF therapy.

3.3.1.1 Focal/grid laser

According to the Early Treatment Diabetes Retinopathy Study (EDTRS), focal/grid macular laser was shown to be effective in marked macular edema reduction or cure, in addition to the reduction of the risk of moderate visual loss by 50% at the termination of the 3-year follow-up trial [56]. More recent clinical trials following ETDRS showed a similar result of reduction of moderate visual loss by 50% with a gain of ≥10 letters of visual acuity in 28% of DME eyes [57].

Focal laser applied to leaking microaneurysms at least 300–500 μm from the center of the macula and guided by FA in noncenter-involving DME remains a gold standard for treatment of this subset of DME [43, 58].

In grid laser, mild power laser marks are made with a spot size of 50 μm to 200 μm, to treat widespread and diffuse edema [59], particularly in cases of resistance or contraindication to the use of anti-VEGF drugs [60].

Combining laser photocoagulation with anti-VEGF injections for DME has been described in several studies. Combined treatment was found to be more effective in improving visual acuity in DME patients. With combined treatment, 10 to 40% of patients gained ≥15 letters in their VA [61–63].

The mechanism of action of focal/grid photocoagulation is not clear, although direct closure of leaking microaneurysms in focal laser and the destruction of the high oxygen consuming photoreceptors, reduction of retinal tissue and improvement of oxygenation together with restoration of the function of retinal pigment epithelial cells in grid laser are postulated mechanisms [64–66] (**Figure 9**).

3.3.1.2 Micropulse laser

The basis of micropulse laser (diode laser 810 μm and yellow laser 577 μm) unlike the conventional continuous-wave laser is to apply the minimum laser irradiance (watts per square meter). The aim is to raise the temperature of the RPE cells leading

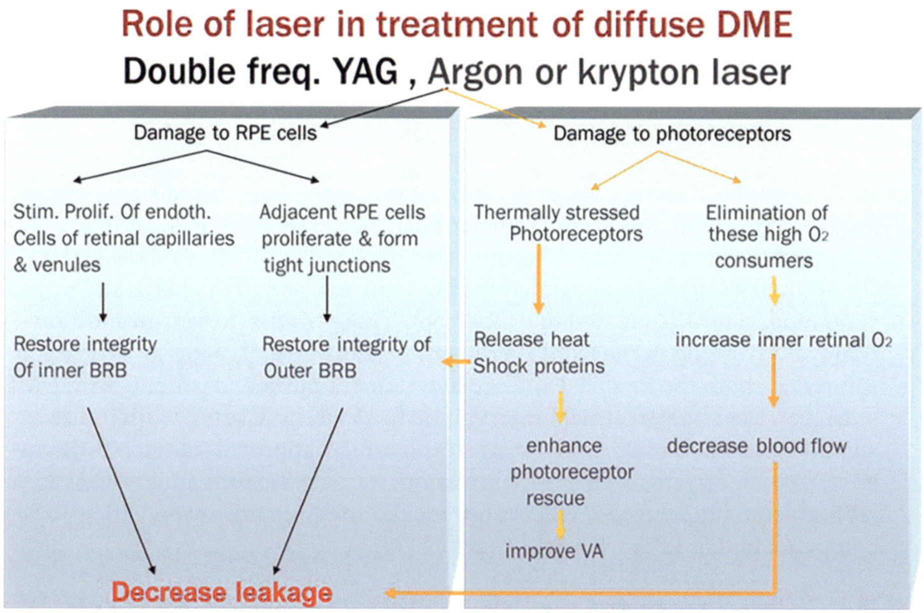

Figure 9.
Possible mechanism of action of grid laser in the management of DME.

to their activation, but without exceeding the protein denaturation threshold in the neural retina which is thus not injured by the laser application.

In the traditional continuous-wave mode, the preset laser energy is delivered totally in a single laser pulse of 0.1–0.5 s. In the micropulse mode, a train of repetitive short laser pulses (each pulse is 100–300 μs) is delivered within an envelope of laser energy having a width of 0.1–0.5 s [67].

The Diabetic Macular Edema and Diode Subthreshold Micropulse Laser (DIAMONDS) trial found that the subthreshold micropulse laser was noninferior to the traditional continuous-wave laser (focal/grid) in terms of functional (VA improvement) and anatomical (optical coherence tomography central macular thickness (OCT CMT)) improvement [68].

3.3.2 Anti-VEGF drugs

The two anti-VEGF drugs Food and Drug Administration (FDA) approved and most commonly used are ranibizumab and aflibercept.

1. *Ranibizumab*: (Lucentis®, Genentech, South San Francisco, CA, USA/Roche, Basel, Switzerland) Ranibizumab was the first FDA-approved anti-VEGF. It is a humanized monoclonal antibody that acts by interrupting the functions of VEGF isoforms [43].

2. *Aflibercept*: (Eylea®, Regeneron, Tarrytown, NY, USA) [69]. Aflibercept is a 115-kDa, glycosylated, recombinant, fusion protein with native vascular endothelial growth factor receptor (VEGFR) ligand-binding sequences attached

to the fragment crystallizable (Fc) segment of a human immunoglobulin G1 (IgG1). Aflibercept differs from the other anti-VEGF drugs, in that in addition to its binding capability to all isoforms of vascular endothelial growth factor A (VEGF-A) and vascular endothelial growth factor B (VEGF-B), it also binds to placental growth factor (PlGF) [70].

3. *Brolucizumab*: (Beovu®; Novartis) Brolucizumab is a humanized single-chain antibody fragment, and it is the smallest functional subunit of an antibody approved for intravitreal use. Results from recent phase III trials showed the superior efficacy of brolucizumab in both reducing retinal thickness and retinal fluid reduction as compared to Aflibercept. Those results present an additional therapeutic option in the DME treatment. In addition to its superior efficacy, it can reduce both the financial and social treatment burden in patients with DME with increased intertreatment intervals up to 16 weeks. Caution with its use should be taken, however, regarding the post-FDA-approval side effects discovered, particularly intraocular inflammation, retinal vasculitis and retinal vascular occlusion (an increased risk for intraocular inflammatory events (0.3–4.7% compared to 0.6–1.7% with Aflibercept)) [71].

4. *Bevacizumab*: (Avastin®, Genentech, South San Francisco, CA, USA/Roche, Basel, Switzerland) Bevacizumab is FDA-approved only to treat local and metastatic solid cancers but because of its cheaper price and treatment efficiency, it has been used off-label for treatment of DME [72, 73]. It is a high-affinity, 149-kDa, recombinant, humanized, full-length murine antibody that binds all isoforms of VEGF-A. Being a cheaper alternative, it is extensively used off-label as an intravitreal injection for the treatment of DME [73, 74].

5. *Faricimab*: Faricimab is a bi-specific antibody, i.e., a single molecule that functions by a dual mechanism, and it has the advantage of blocking both angiopoietin-2 (Ang-2) and VEGF-A. (Ang-2) is an antagonist to endothelial receptor tyrosine kinase (Tie2) (**Figure 3**), when blocked, the vascular structure is stabilized inhibiting continuous loss of pericytes with less inflammation [75, 76].

In the BOULEVARD trial, the patients who received 6.0 mg of faricimab did not need frequent re-treatments as compared to the group of patients who received ranibizumab [77].

In the YOSEMITE and RHINE trials, faricimab administered at 8- and at 16-week intervals was not inferior to Aflibercept administered every 8 weeks as regards visual improvement [78–81].

Several studies compared the efficacy of anti-VEGF drugs and laser treatment:

In all trials comparing Ranibizumab with sham injection (RESOLVE, RISE and RIDE), or with laser treatment (READ-2 and RESTORE), or in association with prompt and deferred laser (DRCR.net Protocol I), it was proved that Ranibizumab had better outcomes as compared to laser treatment for DME.

Similarly, studies with Aflibercept as DA VINCI (DME and VEGF trap-eye: investigation of clinical impact), Vision Impairment due to DME (VIVID-DME) and Study of Intravitreal Aflibercept Injection in Patients with Diabetic Macular Edema (VISTA-DME), also proved a better response with Aflibercept as compared to laser in the management of DME [82].

3.3.3 Steroids

1. *Triamcinolone acetonide (TA):* Intravitreal triamcinolone acetonide has not yet been approved for DME, however, in several studies its intravitreal use provided good visual acuity and anatomical improvements [83–85].

In pseudophakic eyes, the efficacy of Triamcinolone acetonide combined with laser therapy was found to be comparable to that of combined ranibizumab and laser therapy [86, 87].

The high incidence of glaucoma (about 44%) and cataract development (about 54%) make its use unsatisfactory [86, 87].

2. *Dexamethasone intravitreal implant (DEX implant; Ozurdex; Allergan, Inc., Irvine, CA, USA):*

OZURDEX® (dexamethasone intravitreal implant) 0.7 mg is a biodegradable implant injected into the vitreous to treat diabetic macular edema. Ozurdex was approved for treatment of diabetic macular edema in late 2014 [88].

In the MEAD trials, a great percentage of patients achieved a visual gain of ≥15-letters from baseline with improved central retinal thickness (CRT) by OCT [89].

In the PLACID trial, comparing Ozurdex monotherapy to laser monotherapy, a higher percentage of patients treated with dexamethasone achieved at least 10 letters better improvement as compared to those treated with laser monotherapy [90].

Dexamethasone has lower lipophilic properties than other corticosteroids, with consequent lower binding affinity to the trabecular meshwork. Thus, dexamethasone implants are associated with lower risks of glaucoma and cataract as compared to other steroids used for treatment of DME [91].

3. *Fluocinolone acetonide (FA) intravitreal implant:* It is a nonerodible implant approved for the treatment of diabetic macular edema (DME). The injectable intravitreal implant releases fluocinolone acetonide at a rate of about 0.2 μg/day for a duration of about 36 months [92].

The Fluocinolone Acetonide in Diabetic Macular Edema (FAME) trials showed that, in patients with center-involved DME previously treated with laser photocoagulation, FA intravitreal implant was superior as compared to sham injection in improving VA more than 15 letters at 24 months and at 36 months [93, 94].

The two commonest side effects of the drug were cataract (86%) and nearly all of them required cataract extraction and intraocular pressure (IOP) elevation (37%). Raised IOP was mostly treated with antiglaucoma medications, with <5% of eyes requiring glaucoma surgery [95].

3.4 Guidelines for treatment

3.4.1 Subclinical DME (SCME)

Subclinical macular edema is defined as thickening of the center of the macula identified by OCT but not detected on clinical examination [96].

Monitoring the progression of subclinical DME (SCME), the Diabetic Retinopathy Clinical Research Network (DRCR.net) showed that about a quarter to half of eyes would progress to clinically significant macular edema (CSME) within 2 years, and are 12 times more prone to the development of CSME as compared to eyes without SCME, particularly if there is increased retinal thickening within the outer ring of the ETDRS grid. This is an important indicator that SCME is an important biomarker for development of center-involving diabetic macular edema (CIME) and this was also found to be commoner in female patients [96, 97].

On the other hand, there is a controversy as to whether the level of HBA1c is related to the progression of SCME to CIME or not [97, 98].

The management of subclinical DME is mainly the prevention of its progression to CSME. Scheduled follow-up visits, with OCT performed together with glycemic control, and strict control of the other systemic risk factors mentioned above are recommended [43].

3.4.2 Treatment recommendations for non-center-involving DME (non-CIME)

Noncenter-involving DME represents a precursor to the development of center-involved clinically significant ME. If not treated, it was found that 38% of eyes will gain at least 50 μm in CMT over 2 years [96].

Laser treatment is recommended for this subset of DME by most authors.

A modified ETDRS (mETDRS) laser treatment was recommended by the Diabetic Retinopathy Clinical Research (DRCR) net study and was based on treating areas of thickened macula (as shown by OCT imaging) and areas of nonperfusion (detected by OCTA and FA) and leaking microaneurysm (detected by FA) with less intense and smaller burns than in the original ETDRS treatment. Results of this study showed a gain of 15 letters in 25% of the patients [99]. Complications of this technique however include central scotomata and loss of central vision caused by progressive enlargement of the laser scars [100].

Focal laser is another option adopted where focal laser is applied to all leaking microaneurysms 500–3000 μm away from the fovea. Results of this line of treatment showed improvement of visual acuity (VA) in 21% of eyes and stabilization of baseline VA in 61% of eyes [101].

One study, however, recommended either observation until involvement of the center of the macula or alternatively initiating anti-VEGF therapy or focal laser photocoagulation [58].

3.4.3 Treatment recommendations for center-involved DME

Most of the guidelines for center-involved DME recommend anti-VEGF intravitreal injections as the first line of treatment, unless contraindicated as in cases of a recent cardiovascular or cerebrovascular event within the previous 3–6 months, breast feeding and pregnancy [43, 58, 102–104].

Anti-VEGF injection is currently loaded by following one of the following protocols:

1. Treat and extend protocol (T&E)

With Ranibizumab, after the initial 3-monthly loading doses, the patient is switched to a T&E regimen if there were no signs of disease activity as indicated by

OCT images and the best-corrected visual acuity (BCVA) was either the same or better as compared to that at the last visit. In this regimen, follow-up visits were extended by a 4-week interval so long as there was no disease activity for a maximum duration of 24 weeks. If signs of activity appeared (recurrence of intraretinal or subretinal fluid or CRT more than 300 μm), a new injection is given and the follow-up duration is shortened by 4 weeks to a minimum interval of 4 weeks between the visits [105].

For aflibercept, the recommended regimen is five loading monthly injections followed by one injection every 2 months for the first year. Once stabilized, the duration could be extended as above [106].

2. Pro re nata (PRN) regimen

In this regimen, the patient received the usual loading dose followed by monthly injections until there was no disease activity by OCT and the best-corrected visual acuity (BCVA) was either stabilized or improved as compared to the previous visit. Patients then were scheduled for regular follow-ups every 1–3 months and received no further injections, unless recurrence of disease activity was noted on OCT [105].

In a recent meta-analysis comparing T&E and PRN protocols for DME, there was no clear advantage in reducing the number of injections between the two groups; however, there were, in the T&E regimen, limited gains in visual and anatomical outcomes. The T&E regimen also allows for fewer patient visits, thereby reducing treatment burden [107].

All guidelines agree that nonresponders to anti-VEGF treatment (after the first 3–6 injections) should be switched to another anti-VEGF or to steroids. The definition of (nonresponders), however, differed in various guidelines. In one *post hoc* analysis exploring the relationship between early retinal anatomical (CMT on OCT imaging) and functional (visual acuity) responses (after 12 weeks) and long-term same anatomical and visual outcomes (weeks 52 and 156) in eyes treated with ranibizumab plus prompt or deferred laser (in Protocol I study), a conclusion was set that a reduction of less than 20% in central retinal thickness or less than 5-letter improvement in VA is to be categorized as (nonresponder) [108, 109].

The criteria of (nonresponders) in the American Delphi Panel guidelines were however different, they considered that failure to achieve a visual acuity of 20/40 or better or failure to achieve a reduction of at least 50% of excess macular thickness on OCT after the initial 3–6-month loading dose is to be considered nonresponsiveness [102].

The Spanish Delphi panel also had different criteria for nonresponders. They considered a less than 10% reduction in CRT or a less than 5 letter improvement in VA a criterion for nonresponsiveness [103].

For nonresponders, a switch to another anti-VEGF is recommended if the patient is phakic, to lower the incidence of cataract and glaucoma development. If the DME remained without responding, a switch to steroids is recommended [43]. Dexamethasone implant is the first choice in the steroid group followed by fluocinolone acetonide intravitreal implant in case of steroid nonresponsiveness [110].

A steroid dexamethasone implant (DEX implant; Ozurdex) can be used as a first-line treatment if anti-VEGF is contraindicated, in the above-mentioned conditions, or if there is poor compliance with the anti-VEGF regimen (because of the frequent visits or social or economic issues), and may also be recommended in patients who are vitrectomized, pseudophakic (because cataract development is not now an issue) or with chronic DME [111, 112]. IOP measurement and monitoring the development of cataract should be regularly checked in patients in whom a steroid implant is used [112].

One study suggested that DME associated with an increased inflammatory response, especially the cystoid and the sensory neural detachment types, as mentioned above, may resolve better with steroids as compared to anti-VEGFs [14].

3.4.3.1 Management of center-involved DME in pregnancy

Early Diabetic Treatment Retinopathy Study (ETDRS) recommended the use of grid or focal laser for clinically significant macular edema (CSME) in general. This was, however, before the era of anti-VEGFs and steroids [113]. ETDRS guidelines were, however, not specific for pregnancy, but two studies [114, 115] supported the use of macular laser at the earliest to prevent irreversible damage. Another study [116] recommended the use of micropulse laser for foveal involvement, as it is safer.

Anti-VEGF and triamcinolone are better to be avoided during pregnancy for fear of teratogenicity in cases where there is refractory DME. Since steroids were proven to be more effective in improving VA after 4 months of follow-up as compared to laser as proved by the Diabetic Retinopathy Clinical Research (DRCR) Network [117], it is therefore recommended to use dexamethasone implant for DME that developed before pregnancy [43].

Observation is a reasonable management option for pregnant patients with mild diabetic macular edema (DME) or DME developing during pregnancy since the edema may well resolve after delivery [43, 118].

The American Academy of Ophthalmology Preferred Practice Patterns recommend that pregnant diabetic patients undergo dilated fundus examination in the first trimester, with subsequent follow-up determined by the severity of retinopathy, as per every 3–6 months for moderate nonproliferative diabetic retinopathy (NPDR) and those with severe NPDR or worse should be examined every 1–3 months. *Postpartum* follow-up should continue during the first year [117].

3.4.3.2 Management of diabetic macular edema associated with proliferative diabetic retinopathy

In patients with noncenter-involved DME associated with PDR, a focal laser is a good option to be used to treat the DME [119].

If the PDR is presented with center-involved DME, anti-VEGF therapy is recommended, it will improve the DME and cause regression of the neovascularization, then, PRP can be applied. Both ranibizumab and aflibercept were equally effective in improving visual acuity and reducing CRT in eyes with DME and PDR after 2 years; however, the number of microaneurysms, supplementary laser PRP and micropulse laser sessions were higher in the Ranibizumab group [120].

3.4.3.3 Surgical management of DME

Currently, the indication of pars plana vitrectomy (PPV) in eyes with DME is the presence of vitreomacular traction or the persistence of macular edema following intensive intravitreal injection with anti-VEGF or steroids [121, 122].

The performance of internal limiting membrane (ILM) peeling is, however, a matter of controversy. Complications from ILM peeling in cases of DME when the retinal architecture is disorganized and weakened by a longstanding and chronic DME, such as rupturing intraretinal cystoid spaces, might be expected. In one study, the functional results as regards improvement of VA did not differ whether the ILM was peeled or not [122].

As regards the preoperative OCT findings, it was found that eyes with neurosensory detachment had the best postoperative VA improvement following PPV, while eyes with sponge-like diffuse retinal thickening (SDRT) did not show any VA improvement following PPV [123].

Although from the theoretical point of view, PPV reduces VEGF and other DME-promoting cytokine concentration in the premacular area [124] and increases oxygen supply to the ischemic retina further suppressing VEGF production with consequent reduction of DME, yet there is no universal agreement in the performance of PPV for cases of DME without traction [125, 126].

Results of clinical trials appear controversial [121–123]. Although a limited improvement of function and a short-term improvement in macular thickness reduction following surgery were reported by some authors [121, 127], others demonstrated a significant benefit [128, 129].

3.4.3.4 Cataract extraction in the presence of DME

It is usually recommended to give anti-VEGF 1–2 weeks before cataract extraction to stabilize DME prior to surgery. A less preferred option is to give the anti-VEGF during the surgery [130, 131].

3.5 Newer advances to solve the unmet needs in the management of DME

1. Predictive medicine:

This subset of medicine detects the occurrence of a disease before its manifestations appear in an individual, as per population-based cross-sectional studies linked to clinical data. People at risk can therefore have personalized treatment plans with better treatment outcomes [132, 133].

2. Solving the problems of delayed diagnosis, referral and screening

    a. The advent of new nonmydriatic ultrawide field fundus cameras to facilitate examination and documentation through miotic pupils [134].

    b. The use of handheld devices to facilitate screening and is also cost effective [135].

    c. The use of artificial intelligence (AI) to analyze the fundus photographs can overcome the deficiency of healthcare workers [136].

    d. Measuring the level of retinal flavoprotein fluorescence, which was found to be elevated in diabetic eyes with retinopathy, as compared to diabetic eyes without retinopathy. This was recently introduced using a noninvasive imaging machine [137].

3. Reducing the burden of monthly anti-VEGF injections

A Ranibizumab port delivery system, which is a sustained delivery refillable implant, is described in ongoing studies for approval. It can be implanted over the pars plana without sutures. It is now in phase II trial (LADDER, ClinicalTrials.gov identifier: NCT02510794) [135].

4. Overcoming the poor response to anti-VEGFs:

Newer pathway drugs are recently under investigation for the treatment of DME (**Table 3**).

Agent	Mechanism of action	Route of administration	Current development status
Pharmacological agents targeting the angioprotein/Tie pathway [138]			
Razuprotafib (AKB-9778)	Small-molecule inhibitor of VE-PTP	Subcutaneous injection	Completed phase 2 for DME and DR
Nesvacumab	Fully human IgG1 monoclonal antibody inhibiting Ang-2	Intravitreal injection as a co-formulation with aflibercept	Completed phase 2 for DME development currently discontinued
Faricimab (Vabysmo)	Bispecific IgG1-based antibody inhibiting both Ang-2 and VEGF simultaneously	Intravitreal injection	Completed phases 2 and 3 for DME and nAMD. Approved by the US FDA for the treatment of DME and nAMD
AXT107	Type IV collagen-derived peptide that activates Tie-2 and inhibits VEGF-A and VEGF-C	Intravitreal injection	Ongoing phase 1/2a for DME and nAMD
Pharmacologic agents with an anti-inflammatory action: [139]			
APX3330	Redox factor-1 (Ref-1) inhibition; can potentially reduce proinflammatory and hypoxic signaling	Small-molecule oral tablet	Phase 2
LKA651	Erythropoietin inhibitor	Intravitreal injection	Phase 2
Endothelial dysfunction blockers: [139]			
AR-13503	Active metabolite of netarsudil and inhibitor of Rho kinase (ROCK) and protein kinase C (PKC)	Implant	Phase 1
CU06–1004	Inhibitor of vascular leakage and inflammation, as shown in various animal models	Oral capsule	Phase 1
THR-149	Bicyclic peptide inhibitor targeting plasma kallikrein AAV8 vector	Intravitreal injection	Phase 2
Gene therapy [139]			
RGX-314	AAV8 vector containing a transgene for anti-VEGF fab	Intravitreal injection	Phase 2

Table 3.
Recently, pathway drugs under investigation are used for the treatment of DME.

4. Conclusion

Diabetes mellitus (DM) and its complications are a major public health burden worldwide. Diabetic macular edema is a vision-threatening complication of DR and a major cause of vision loss in diabetic patients.

The pathogenesis of diabetic macular edema is very diverse and consequently, the results of treatment are sometimes not satisfactory. Available treatment options include retinal laser photocoagulation, antivascular endothelial growth factor (anti-VEGF) agents, intravitreal corticosteroids and vitreoretinal surgery.

More drug options utilizing different pharmacologic pathways are now being investigated to improve the visual results posttreatment and decrease the economic and social burden the patients are experiencing.

Conflict of interest

"The author declares no conflict of interest."

Author details

Ahmed Darwish
Faculty of Medicine, Ophthalmology, Ain Shams University, Egypt

*Address all correspondence to: ahmed_darwish33@hotmail.com

References

[1] Williams R et al. Epidemiology of diabetic retinopathy and macular oedema: A systematic review. Eye. 2004;**18**(10):963-983

[2] Yau JW et al. Global prevalence and major risk factors of diabetic retinopathy. Diabetes Care. 2012;**35**(3):556-564

[3] Zhang X et al. Prevalence of diabetic retinopathy in the United States, 2005-2008. Journal of the American Medical Association. 2010;**304**(6):649-656

[4] Ruta LM. Prevalence of diabetic retinopathy in type 2 diabetes in developing and developed countries. Diabetic Medicine. 2013;**30**(4):387-398

[5] Das A, McGuire PG, Rangasamy S. Diabetic macular edema: Pathophysiology and novel therapeutic targets. Ophthalmology. 2015;**122**:1375-1394

[6] Battagliaa MP. A Pathogenetic classification of diabetic macular edema. Ophthalmic Research. 2018;**60**(1):23-28. DOI: 10.1159/000484350

[7] Antonetti DA, Barber AJ, Bronson SK, et al. JDRF diabetic retinopathy center group. Diabetic retinopathy: Seeing beyond glucose-induced microvascular disease. Diabetes. 2006;**55**:2401-2411

[8] Vujosevic S et al. Early microvascular and neural changes in patients with type 1 and type 2 diabetes mellitus without clinical signs of diabetic retinopathy. Retina. 2019;**39**:435-445

[9] Daruich A, Matet AM, et al. Mechanisms of macular edema: Beyond the surface. Progress in Retinal and Eye Research. 2018;**63**:20-68

[10] Klaassen I et al. Molecular basis of the inner blood-retinal barrier and its breakdown in diabetic macular edema and other pathological conditions. Progress in Retinal and Eye Research. 2013;**34**:19-48

[11] Benveniste N. Immune function of astrocytes. Glia. 2001;**36**(2):180-190

[12] Sun K, Stitt AW. Diabetic retinopathy: Current understanding, mechanisms, and treatment strategies. JCI Insight. 2017;**2**(14):e93751

[13] Checchin D. Potential role of microglia in retinal blood vessel formation. Investigative Ophthalmology & Visual Science. 2006;**47**(8):3595-3602

[14] Yoo-Ri Chung R et al. Review article role of inflammation in classification of diabetic macular edema by optical coherence tomography. Journal of Diabetes Research. 2019;**2019**:8164250, 8 pages. DOI: 10.1155/2019/8164250

[15] Simo R. The retinal pigment epithelium: Something more than a constituent of the blood-retinal barrier—implications for the pathogenesis of diabetic retinopathy. Journal of Biomedicine & Biotechnology. 2010;**2010**:190724, 15 pages

[16] Arroba AI, Valverde AM. Modulation of microglia in the retina: New insights into diabetic retinopathy. Acta Diabetologica. 2017;**54**(6):527-533

[17] Darwish A. Hyper-reflective spots in OCT imaging in retinal disease: Imaging features and clinic-pathologic correlation. New Advances in Medicine and Medical Science. 2023;**1**:47-55. DOI: 10.9734/bpi/namms/v1/5665E

[18] Bolz M, Schmidt-Erfurth U, Deak G, et al. Optical coherence tomographic hyperreflective foci: A morphologic sign of lipid extravasation in diabetic macular edema. Ophthalmology. 2009;**116**:914-920

[19] Uji A, Murakami T, Nishijima K, et al. Association between hyperreflective foci in the outer retina, status of photoreceptor layer, and visual acuity in diabetic macular edema. American Journal of Ophthalmology. 2012;**153**:710-717 717. e1

[20] Framme C, Schweizer P, Imesch M, et al. Behavior of SD-OCT-detected hyperreflective foci in the retina of antiVEGF-treated patients with diabetic macular edema. Investigative Ophthalmology & Visual Science. 2012;**53**:5814-5818

[21] Tang J, Kern TS. Inflammation in diabetic retinopathy. Progress in Retinal and Eye Research. 2011;**30**(5):343-358

[22] Spaide RF. Retinal vascular cystoid macular edema: Review and new theory. Retina. 2016;**36**(10):1823-1842

[23] Bringmann A et al. Müller cells in the healthy and diseased retina. Progress in Retinal and Eye Research. 2006;**25**(4):397-424

[24] Ascaso FJ. The role of inflammation in the pathogenesis of macular edema secondary to retinal vascular diseases. Mediators of Inflammation. 2014;**2014**:432685, 6 pages

[25] Eichler W. Angiogenesis-related factors derived from retinal glial (Müller) cells in hypoxia. Neuroreport. 2004;**15**(10):1633-1637

[26] Portillo JC et al. CD40 in retinal Müller cells induces P2X7-dependent cytokine expression in macrophages/microglia in diabetic mice and development of early experimental diabetic retinopathy. Diabetes. 2017;**66**(2):483-493

[27] Huang H, He J, Johnson D, Wei Y, Liu Y, Wang S, et al. Deletion of placental growth factor prevents diabetic retinopathy and is associated with Akt activation and HIF1alpha-VEGF pathway inhibition. Diabetes. 2015;**64**:200-212

[28] Lupo G, Motta C, Giurdanella G, Anfuso CD, Alberghina M, Drago F, et al. Role of phospholipases A2 in diabetic retinopathy: In vitro and in vivo studies. Biochemical Pharmacology. 2013;**86**:1603-1613

[29] Antonetti DA, Barber AJ, Hollinger LA, Wolpert EB, Gardner TW. Vascular endothelial growth factor induces rapid phosphorylation of tight junction proteins occludin and zonula occluden 1. A potential mechanism for vascular permeability in diabetic retinopathy and tumors. The Journal of Biological Chemistry. 1999;**274**:23463-23467

[30] Rousseau S, Houle F, Landry J, Huot J. p 38 MAP kinase activation by vascular endothelial growth factor mediates actin reorganization and cell migration in human endothelial cells. Oncogene. 1997;**15**:2169-2177

[31] Rangasamy S, Srinivasan R, Maestas J, McGuire PG, Das A. A potential role for angiopoietin 2 in the regulation of the blood-retinal barrier in diabetic retinopathy. Investigative Ophthalmology and Visual Science. 2011;**52**:3784-3791

[32] Nishikawa T, Edelstein D, Du XL, et al. Normalizing mitochondrial superoxide production blocks three pathways of hyperglycaemic damage. Nature. 2000;**404**(6779):787-790

[33] Mustapha NM. Research article. NADPH oxidase versus mitochondria – Derived ROS in glucose induced apoptosis of pericytes in early diabetic retinopathy. Journal of Ophthalmology. 2010;**2010**:746978, 10 pages. DOI: 10.1155/2010/746978

[34] Brandes RP, Kreuzer J. Vascular NADPH oxidases: Molecular mechanisms of activation. Cardiovascular Research. 2005;**65**(1):16-27

[35] Fujiwara A. En face image-based classification of diabetic macular edema using swept source optical coherence tomography. Science Reports. 2021;**11**:7665 Available from: www.nature.com/scientificreports. DOI: 10.1038/s41598-021-87440-3

[36] Makita S, Hong Y, Yamanari M, et al. Optical coherence angiography. Optics Express. 2006;**14**:7821-7840

[37] American Academy of Ophthalmology, Retina/Vitreous Panel. Diabetic Retinopathy Preferred Practice Pattern Guidelines. Chicago: American Academy of Ophthalmology, Retina/Vitreous Panel; 2019

[38] Panozzo G et al. An optical coherence tomography-based grading of diabetic maculopathy proposed by an international expert panel: The European School for Advanced Studies in ophthalmology classification. European Journal of Ophthalmology. 2019;**30**:1-11. DOI: 10.1177/112067211988039

[39] Gerendas B et al. Morphological parameters relevant for the visual and anatomic outcomes during anti-VEGF therapy of diabetic macular edema in the RESTORE trial. Investigative Ophthalmology & Visual Science. 2014;**55**:1791

[40] Sun JK et al. Disorganization of the retinal inner layers as a predictor of visual acuity in eyes with center-involved diabetic macular edema. JAMA Ophthalmology. 2014;**132**:1309-1316

[41] Shin HJ et al. Association between photoreceptor integrity and visual outcome in diabetic macular edema. Graefe's Archive for Clinical and Experimental Ophthalmology. 2012;**250**:61-70

[42] Rayees N et al. Baseline choroid thickness as a predictor for response to anti-VEGF therapy in diabetic macular edema. American Journal of Ophthalmology. 2015;**159**:85-91

[43] AlQahtani A et al. Saudi Arabia guidelines for diabetic macular edema: A consensus of the Saudi retina group, clinical practice guidelines. Saudi Medical Journal. 2021;**42**(2):131-145

[44] The Diabetes Control and Complications Trial Research Group. The effect of intensive treatment of diabetes on the development and progression of long-term complications in insulin-dependent diabetes mellitus. The New England Journal of Medicine. 1993;**329**:977-986

[45] Diabetes Control and Complications Trial Research Group. The relationship of glycemic exposure (HbA1c) to the risk of development and progression of retinopathy in the diabetes control and complications trial. Diabetes. 1995;**44**:968-983

[46] UK Prospective Diabetes Study (UKPDS) Group. Effect of intensive blood-glucose control with metformin on complications in overweight patients with type 2 diabetes (UKPDS 34). Lancet. 1998;**352**:854-865

[47] Writing Team for the Diabetes Control and Complications Trial/Epidemiology of Diabetes Interventions and Complications Research Group. Effect of intensive therapy on the microvascular complications of type 1 diabetes mellitus. JAMA. 2002;**287**(19):2563-2569. DOI: 10.1001/jama.287.19.2563

[48] Chew EY, Ambrosius WT, Davis MD, et al. Effects of medical therapies on retinopathy progression in type 2 diabetes. The New England Journal of Medicine. 2010;**363**:233-244

[49] Saudek CD. Non-ophthalmologic findings of the diabetes control and complications trial. Survey of Ophthalmology. 1995;**40**(2):157-162. DOI: 10.1016/s0039-6257(95)80005-0

[50] Christine A et al. Medical management and prevention and treatment of diabetic macular edema. Survey of Ophthalmology. 2013;**58**(5):459-465. DOI: 10.1016/j.survophthal.2012.10.002

[51] Davis MD, Fisher MR, Gangnon RE, et al. Risk factors for high-risk proliferative diabetic retinopathy and severe visual loss: Early treatment diabetic retinopathy study report #18. Investigative Ophthalmology & Visual Science. 1998;**39**:233-252

[52] Klein R, Klein BE, Moss SE, Davis MD, DeMets DL. Glycosylated hemoglobin predicts the incidence and progression of diabetic retinopathy. Journal of the American Medical Association. 1988;**260**:2864-2871

[53] The Diabetes Control and Complications Trial group. The effect of intensive diabetes treatment on the progression of diabetic retinopathy in insulin dependent diabetes mellitus. Archives of Ophthalmology. 1995;**113**:36-51

[54] Lopes-Virella MF, Baker NL, Hunt KJ, et al. High concentrations of AGE-LDL and oxidized LDL in circulating immune complexes are associated with progression of retinopathy in type 1 diabetes. Diabetes Care. 2012;**35**:1333-1340

[55] International Diabetes Federation. Clinical Practice Recommendations for Managing Diabetic Macular Edema. Brussels, Belgium: International Diabetes Federation; 2019

[56] Early Treatment Diabetic Retinopathy Study Research Group. Treatment techniques and clinical guidelines for photocoagulation of diabetic macular edema. Early treatment diabetic retinopathy study report number 2. Ophthalmology. 1987;**94**:761-774

[57] Elman MJ et al. Randomized trial evaluating ranibizumab plus prompt or deferred laser or triamcinolone plus prompt laser for diabetic macular edema. Ophthalmology. 2010;**117**(6): 1064-1077.e35

[58] Qassimi N et al. Management of Diabetic Macular Edema: Guidelines from the emirates Society of Ophthalmology. Ophthalmology and Therapy. 2022;**11**:1937-1950. DOI: 10.1007/s40123-022-00547-2

[59] Romero-Aroca P, Reyes-Torres J, Baget-Bernaldiz M, Blasco-Sune C. Laser treatment for diabetic macular edema in the 21st century. Current Diabetes Reviews. 2014;**10**:100-112

[60] Browning DJ, Stewart MW, Lee C. Diabetic macular edema: Evidence-based management. Indian Journal of Ophthalmology. 2018;**66**:1736-1750

[61] Mitchell P, Bandello F, Schmidt-Erfurth U, Lang GE, Massin P, Schlingemann RO, et al. The RESTORE study: Ranibizumab monotherapy or combined with laser versus laser monotherapy for diabetic macular edema. Ophthalmology. 2011;**118**:615-625

[62] Elman MJ, Aiello LP, Beck RW, Bressler NM, Bressler SB, Edwards AR, et al. Randomized trial evaluating ranibizumab plus prompt or deferred laser or triamcinolone plus prompt laser for diabetic macular edema. Ophthalmology. 2010;**117**:1064-1077

[63] Michaelides M, Kaines A, Hamilton RD, Fraser-Bell S, Rajendram R, Quhill F, et al. A prospective randomized trial of intravitreal bevacizumab or laser therapy in the management of diabetic macular edema (BOLT study). 12-month data: Report 2. Ophthalmology. 2010;**117**:1078-1086

[64] Arnarsson A, Stefansson E. Laser treatment and the mechanism of edema reduction in branch retinal vein occlusion. Investigative Ophthalmology and Visual Science. 2000;**41**:877-879

[65] Ogata N, Tombran-Tink J, Jo N, Mrazek D, Matsumura M. Upregulation of pigment epithelium-derived factor after laser photocoagulation. American Journal of Ophthalmology. 2001;**132**:427-429

[66] Tutela GA, Zarbin MA. Diabetic macular edema: Pathogenesis and treatment. Survey of Ophthalmology. 2009;**54**(1):1-32

[67] Lanzetta P, Dorin G, Pirracchio A, Bandello F. Theoretical bases of non-ophthalmoscopically visible endpoint photocoagulation. Seminars in Ophthalmology. 2001;**16**(1):8-11

[68] Lois N et al. Standard threshold laser versus subthreshold micropulse laser for adults with diabetic macular oedema: The DIAMONDS non-inferiority RCT. Health Technology Assessment. 2022;**26**(50):1-86. DOI: 10.3310/SZKI2484: 10.3310/SZKI2484

[69] Papadopoulos N, Martin J, Ruan Q, et al. Binding and neutralization of vascular endothelial growth factor (VEGF) and related ligands by VEGF trap, ranibizumab and bevacizumab. Angiogenesis. 2012;**15**:171-185

[70] Holash J, Davis S, Papadopoulos N, et al. VEGF-trap: A VEGF blocker with potent antitumor effects. Proceedings of the National Academy of Sciences of the United States of America. 2002;**99**:11393-11398

[71] Blanche LK et al. Brolucizumab for the treatment of diabetic macular edema. Current Opinion in Ophthalmology. 2022;**33**(3):167-173. DOI: 10.1097/ICU.0000000000000849

[72] Low A et al. Comparative effectiveness and harms of intravitreal antivascular endothelial growth factor agents for three retinal conditions: A systematic review and meta-analysis. The British Journal of Ophthalmology. 2019;**103**:442-451. DOI: 10.1136/bjophthalmol-2018-312691

[73] Stewart MW. Anti-VEGF therapy for diabetic macular edema. Current Diabetes Reports. 2014;**14**:510. DOI: 10.1007/s11892-014-0510-4

[74] Jose V et al. Bevacizumab for eye diseases – Legal, regulatory, and ethical overview. Indian Journal of Pharmacology. 2019;**51**(6):377-383. Published online 2020. DOI: 10.4103/ijp.IJP_413_19

[75] Sharma A, Kumar N, Kuppermann BD, Bandello F, Loewenstein A. Faricimab: Expanding horizon beyond VEGF. Eye (London, England). 2020;**34**:802-804

[76] Fuxe J, Tabruyn S, Colton K, Zaid H, Adams A, Baluk P, et al. Pericyte requirement for anti-leak action of angiopoietin-1 and vascular remodeling in sustained inflammation. The American Journal of Pathology. 2011;**178**:2897-2909

[77] Sahni J, Patel SS, Dugel PU, Khanani AM, Jhaveri CD, Wykoff CC, et al. Simultaneous inhibition of angiopoietin-2 and vascular endothelial growth factor-a with faricimab in diabetic macular edema: BOULEVARD phase 2 randomized trial. Ophthalmology. 2019;**126**:1155-1170

[78] File. R data on Roche's faricimab meets primary endpoint and shows strong durability across two global phase III studies for diabetic macular edema, a leading cause of blindness. 2020. Available from: https://www.roche.com/media/releases/medcor-2020-12-21.htm

[79] Roche H-L. A study to evaluate the efficacy and safety of faricimab (RO6867461) in participants with diabetic macular edema (YOSEMITE). NCT03622580. 2018. Available from: https://clinicaltrials.gov/ct2/show/NCT03622593 [Accessed: July 30, 2021]

[80] Roche H-L. A study to evaluate the efficacy and safety of faricimab (RO6867461) in participants with diabetic macular edema (RHINE). NCT03622593. 2018. Available from: https://clinicaltrials.gov/ct2/show/NCT03622593 [Accessed: July 30, 2021]

[81] Iglicki M et al. Next-generation anti-VEGF agents for diabetic macular oedema review article. Eye. 2022;**36**:273-277. DOI: 10.1038/s41433-021-01722-8

[82] Das T, Aurora A, Chhablani J, Giridhar A, Kumar A, Raman R, et al. Evidence-based review of diabetic macular edema management: Consensus statement on Indian treatment guidelines. Indian Journal of Ophthalmology. 2016;**64**:14-25

[83] Zhang Y, Ma J, Meng N, Li H, Qu Y. Comparison of intravitreal triamcinolone acetonide with intravitreal bevacizumab for treatment of diabetic macular edema: A meta-analysis. Current Eye Research. 2013;**38**:578-587

[84] Yolcu Ü, Sobaci G. The effect of combined treatment of bevacizumab and triamcinolone for diabetic macular edema refractory to previous intravitreal mono-injections. International Ophthalmology. 2015;**35**:73-79

[85] Durukan AH, Memisoglu S, Gundogan FC. Is multifocal ERG a reliable index of macular function after triamcinolone acetonide injection in diffuse diabetic macular edema? European Journal of Ophthalmology. 2009;**19**:1017-1027

[86] Elman MJ, Bressler NM, Qin H, Beck RW, Ferris FL, Friedman SM, et al. Expanded 2-year follow-up of ranibizumab plus prompt or deferred laser or triamcinolone plus prompt laser for diabetic macular edema. Ophthalmology. 2011;**118**:609-614

[87] Janet C et al. Intravitreal triamcinolone acetonide for diabetic macular edema. Retina. 2005;**25**(7): 828-834. DOI: 10.1097/00006982-200510000-00002

[88] Retina vitreous associates of Florida: Ozurdex, Ozurdex - Sustained Release

Dexamethasone Implant. Available from: retinavitreous.com

[89] Boyer DS, Yoon YH, Belfort R, Bandello F, Maturi RK, Augustin AJ, et al. Three-year, randomized, sham-controlled trial of dexamethasone intravitreal implant in patients with diabetic macular edema. Ophthalmology. 2014;**121**:1904-1914

[90] Callanan DG, Gupta S, Boyer DS, Ciulla TA, Singer MA, Kuppermann BD, et al. Dexamethasone intravitreal implant in combination with laser photocoagulation for the treatment of diffuse diabetic macular edema. Ophthalmology. 2013;**120**:1843-1851

[91] Cebeci Z, Kir N. Role of implants in the treatment of diabetic macular edema: Focus on the dexamethasone intravitreal implant. Diabetes, Metabolic Syndrome and Obesity. 2015;**8**:555-566

[92] Veritti D et al. Fluocinolone acetonide for the treatment of diabetic macular edema. Expert Opinion on Pharmacotherapy. 2017;**18**(14):1507-1516. DOI: 10.1080/14656566.2017.1363182

[93] Campochiaro PA, Brown DM, Pearson A, et al. Long-term benefit of sustained-delivery fluocinolone acetonide vitreous inserts for diabetic macular edema. Ophthalmology. 2011;**118**:626-635

[94] Campochiaro PA, Brown DM, Pearson A, et al. Sustained delivery fluocinolone acetonide vitreous inserts provide benefit for at least 3 years in patients with diabetic macular edema. Ophthalmology. 2012;**119**:2125-2132

[95] Cunha-Vaz J, Ashton P, Iezzi R, Campochiaro P, Dugel PU, Holz FG, et al. FAME Study Group. Sustained delivery fluocinolone acetonide vitreous implants: Long-term benefit in patients with chronic diabetic macular edema. Ophthalmology. 2014;**121**(10):1892-1903. DOI: 10.1016/j.ophtha.2014.04.019

[96] Bressler NM, Miller KM, Beck RW, Bressler SB, Glassman AR, Schlossman DK. Observational study of subclinical diabetic macular edema. Diabetic Retinopathy Clinical Research Network. Eye (London). 2012;**26**:833-840

[97] Lobo C et al. Subclinical macular edema as a predictor of progression to central-involved macular edema in type 2 diabetes. Ophthalmic Research. 2018;**60**(1):18-22. DOI: 10.1159/000486792Conceição Lobo

[98] Pires I, Santos AR, Nunes S, Lobo C, Cunha Vaz J. Subclinical macular edema as a predictor of progression to clinically significant macular edema in type 2 diabetes. Ophthalmologica. 2013;**230**:201-206

[99] Writing Committee for the Diabetic Retinopathy Clinical Research Network, Fong DS, Strauber SF, Aiello LP, Beck RW, Callanan DG, et al. Comparison of the modified early treatment diabetic retinopathy study and mild macular grid laser photocoagulation strategies for diabetic macular edema. Archives of Ophthalmology. 2007;**125**(4):469-480

[100] Schatz H, Madeira D, McDonald HR, Johnson RN. Progressive enlargement of laser scars following grid laser photocoagulation for diffuse diabetic macular edema. Archives of Ophthalmology. 1991;**109**(11):1549-1551

[101] Perente I. Focal laser photocoagulation in non-center involved diabetic macular edema. Medical Hypothesis Discovery and Innovation in Ophthalmology. Spring, 2014;**3**(1): 9-16

[102] Regillo CD, Callanan DG, Do DV, Fine HF, Holekamp NM, Kuppermann BD, et al. Use of corticosteroids in the treatment of patients with diabetic macular edema who have a suboptimal response to anti-VEGF: Recommendations of an expert panel. Ophthalmic Surgery, Lasers & Imaging Retina. 2017;**48**:291-301

[103] García Layana A, Adán A, Ascaso FJ, Cabrera F, Donate J, Escobar Barranco JJ, et al. Use of intravitreal dexamethasone implants in the treatment of diabetic macular edema: Expert recommendations using a Delphi approach. European Journal of Ophthalmology. 2020;**30**:1042-1052

[104] Giovannini A, Parravano M, Ricci F, Bandello F. Management of diabetic macular edema with intravitreal dexamethasone implants: Expert recommendations using a Delphi-based approach. European Journal of Ophthalmology. 2019;**29**:82-91

[105] Lai T et al. Treat-and-extend vs. pro Re Nata regimen of Ranibizumab for diabetic macular edema—A two-year matched comparative study. Frontiers in Medicine. 2022;**8**:781421. DOI: 10.3389/fmed.2021.781421

[106] Lim SY et al. Treat and extend regimen for diabetic macular oedema-a systematic review and meta-analysis. Graefe's Archive for Clinical and Experimental Ophthalmology. 2023;**261**(2):303-315. DOI: 10.1007/s00417-022-05770-y

[107] Prescriber Guide. Bayer Recommendations for Treatment with Eylea. Prescriber Guide. Leverkusen, Germany: Bayer AG; 2022

[108] Dugel PU et al. Association between early anatomic response to anti-VEGF therapy and long-term outcome in diabetic macular edema. An independent analysis of protocol I study data. Retina. 2018;**39**(1):88-97

[109] Darwish A. Recent trends in the Management of Diabetic Macular Edema, short communication. EC Ophthalmology. 2018;**9**:6

[110] Schmidt-Erfurth U, Garcia-Arumi J, Bandello F, Berg K, Chakravarthy U, Gerendas BS, et al. Guidelines for the management of diabetic macular edema by the European Society of Retina Specialists (EURETINA). Ophthalmologica. 2017;**237**:185-222

[111] Querques G, Darvizeh F, Querques L, et al. Assessment of the real-life usage of intravitreal dexamethasone implant in the treatment of chronic diabetic macular edema in France. Journal of Ocular Pharmacology and Therapeutics. 2016;**32**:383-389

[112] Urbancic M, Gardasevic TI. Dexamethasone implant in the management of diabetic macular edema from clinician's perspective. Clinical Ophthalmology. 2019;**13**:829-840

[113] Photocoagulation for diabetic macular edema. Early Treatment Diabetic Retinopathy Study report number 1. Early Treatment Diabetic Retinopathy Study research group. Arch Ophthalmology. 1985;**103**(12):1796-1806

[114] Rasmussen KL, Laugesen CS, Ringholm L, Vestgaard M, Damm P, Mathiesen ER. Progression of diabetic retinopathy during pregnancy in women with type 2 diabetes. Diabetologia. 2010;**53**:1076-1083

[115] Vestgaard M, Ringholm L, Laugesen CS, Rasmussen KL, Damm P, Mathiesen ER. Pregnancy-induced sight-threatening diabetic retinopathy

in women with type 1 diabetes. Diabetic Medicine. 2010;**27**:431-435

[116] Nicolo M, Musetti D, Traverso CE. Yellow micropulse laser in diabetic macular edema: A short-term pilot study. European Journal of Ophthalmology. 2014;**24**:885-889

[117] Chandrasekaran PR, Madanagopalan VG, Narayanan R. Diabetic retinopathy in pregnancy - a review. Indian Journal of Ophthalmology. 2021;**69**:3015-3025

[118] Rosenthal JM, Johnson MW. Management of Retinal Diseases in pregnant patients, review article. Journal of Ophthalmic and Vision Research. 2018;**13**(1):62-65

[119] Gross J. DRCR.Net prompt PRP vs ranibizumab+deferred PRP for PDR study (protocol S). In: Paper Presented in American Academy of Ophthalmology. Las Vegas; 2015

[120] Hsieh M et al. Diabetic macular edema and proliferative diabetic retinopathy treated with anti-vascular endothelial growth factor under the reimbursement policy in Taiwan. Scientific Reports. 2022;**12**(1):711; Available from: www.nature.com/scientificreports. DOI: 10.1038/s41598-021-04593-x

[121] Hoerauf H, Bruggemann A, Muecke M, et al. Pars plana vitrectomy for diabetic macular edema. Internal limiting membrane delamination vs posterior hyaloid removal. A prospective randomized trial. Graefe's Archive for Clinical and Experimental Ophthalmology. 2011;**249**(7):997-1008

[122] Kumagai K, Hangai M, Ogino N, et al. Effect of internal limiting membrane peeling on long-term visual outcomes for diabetic macular edema. Retina. 2015;**35**(7):1422-1428

[123] Ichiyama Y, Sawada O, Mori T, Fujikawa M, Kawamura H, Ohji M. The effectiveness of vitrectomy for diffuse diabetic macular edema may depend on its preoperative optical coherence tomography pattern. Graefe's Archive for Clinical and Experimental Ophthalmology. 2016;**254**(8):1545-1551

[124] Lee SS, Ghosn C, Yu Z, et al. Vitreous VEGF clearance is increased after vitrectomy. Investigative Ophthalmology & Visual Science. 2010;**51**(4):2135-2138

[125] Stefansson E. Physiology of the vitreous. Graefe's Archive for Clinical and Experimental Ophthalmology. 2009;**247**:147-163

[126] Hagenau F et al. Vitrectomy for diabetic macular edema: Optical coherence tomography criteria and pathology of the Vitreomacular Interface. American Journal of Ophthalmology. 2019;**200**:34-46

[127] Figueroa MS, Contreras I, Noval S. Surgical and anatomical outcomes of pars plana vitrectomy for diffuse non-tractional diabetic macular edema. Retina. 2008;**28**:420-426

[128] Yamamoto T, Naoko A, Takeuchi S. Vitrectomy for diabetic macular edema: The role of posterior vitreous detachment and epimacular membrane. American Journal of Ophthalmology. 2001;**132**(3):369-377

[129] Simunovic MP, Hunyor AP, Ho IV. Vitrectomy for diabetic macular edema: A systematic review and meta-analysis. Canadian Journal of Ophthalmology. 2014;**49**(2):188-195

[130] Boscia F, Giancipoli E, D'Amico Ricci G, Pinna A. Management of macular oedema in diabetic patients undergoing cataract surgery. Current Opinion in Ophthalmology. 2017;**28**:23-28

[131] Baker CW, Almukhtar T, Bressler NM, et al. Macular edema after cataract surgery in eyes without preoperative central-involved diabetic macular edema. JAMA Ophthalmology. 2013;**131**:870-879

[132] Celi LA, Hinske Christian L, Alterovitz G, Szolovits P. An artificial intelligence tool to predict fluid requirement in the intensive care unit: A proof-of-concept study. Critical Care. 2008;**12**(6):R151

[133] Yan W, He M. Predictive medicine in ophthalmology. Ophthalmology. 2017;**124**(4):420-421

[134] Silva PS, Horton MB, Clary D, Lewis DG, Sun JK, Cavallerano JD, et al. Identification of diabetic retinopathy and ungradable image rate with ultrawide field imaging in a National Teleophthalmology Program. Ophthalmology. 2016;**123**(6):1360-1367

[135] Bhattacharjee H, Barman M, Garg M. Diabetic retinopathy and diabetic macular edema: Fighting the emerging global burden. Chapter 20. In: Saxena S, Timothy GC, Lai YY, Sadda SR, editors. Diabetic Macular Edema. Singapore: Springer; 2022. ISBN 978-981-19-7306-2. ISBN 978-981-19-7307-9 (eBook). DOI: 10.1007/978-981-19-7307-9

[136] Bressler NM. Artificial intelligence with deep learning technology looks into diabetic retinopathy screening. Journal of the American Medical Association. 2016;**316**(22):2366-2367

[137] Chen AX, Conti TF, Hom GL, Greenlee TE, Raimondi R, Briskin IN, et al. Functional imaging of mitochondria in retinal diseases using flavoprotein fluorescence. Eye. 2021;**35**(1):74-92

[138] Yip F, LT, Wong CYK, Lai TYY. Agents targeting angiopoietin/tie pathway in diabetic macular edema. Chapter 7. In: Saxena S, Timothy GC, Lai YY, Sadda SR, editors. Diabetic Macular Edema. Singapore: Springer; 2022. ISBN 978-981-19-7306-2. ISBN 978-981-19-7307-9 (eBook). DOI: 10.1007/978-981-19-7307-9

[139] Cabrera AP, Wolinsky EL, Mankad RN, Monickaraj F, Das A. Pathophysiology of diabetic macular edema. Chapter 2. In: Saxena S, Lai GCTYY, Sadda SR, editors. Diabetic Macular Edema. Singapore: Springer; 2022. ISBN 978-981-19-7306-2. ISBN 978-981-19-7307-9 (eBook). DOI: 10.1007/978-981-19-7307-9

Chapter 6

Current Perspective on the Treatment of *Helicobacter pylori* Infection

Malika Taufiq and Maliha Taufiq

Abstract

Helicobacter pylori (*H. pylori*) is a gram-negative aerobic bacteria that infects humans and is responsible for causing more than 80% of cases of chronic gastritis, peptic ulcer disease, and non-cardia gastric cancer. Both peptic ulcer disease and gastric cancer lead to 1 million deaths annually. *H. pylori* is a pathogen responsible for these conditions, highlighting the importance of accurate diagnosis and eradication. Various invasive and non-invasive methods are available to diagnose with varying sensitivity and specificity. Invasive methods include endoscopy, culture, histology, rapid urease test, and molecular tests such as PCR. Non-invasive tests include serology, urea breath test, and stool antigen tests. However, there is growing concern about the increasing resistance of *H. pylori* to commonly available treatments. The lack of availability of invasive and non-invasive procedures to detect *H. pylori* worldwide, particularly in developing countries, are important concerns that need to be addressed in the future. Hence in the future, more emphasis should be placed on the development of an effective vaccine against *H. pylori*.

Keywords: *Helicobacter pylori*, gastric cancer, peptic ulcer disease, triple therapy, resistance, surveillance

1. Introduction

Helicobacter pylori (*H. pylori*) is a gram-negative aerobic bacteria, which was first discovered by Warren and Marshall in 1983. They proved that it can colonize and infect the highly acidic environment of the stomach. Later, they proved that *H. pylori* causes peptic ulcer disease (PUD) [1]. *H. pylori* is a causative agent of acute and chronic gastritis and a major predisposing factor for peptic ulcer disease, gastric cancer, and gastric lymphoma [1]. In 2018, *H. pylori* was responsible for 810,000 new cases of non-cardia gastric cancer worldwide [2], and about 8 in 10 cases of gastric cancer are due to *H. pylori* infection [2]. It infects almost half of the world's population and is almost ubiquitous everywhere. More than 80% of PUD is caused by *H. pylori*, and the estimated lifetime risk of PUD in *H. pylori*-infected patients is approximately 15% [3]. Gastric cancer is the third leading cause of cancer-related death worldwide, and *H. pylori* is responsible for 74.7% of all non-cardia gastric cancer [3]. Gastric cancer and PUD together cause 1 million deaths annually [3]. *Helicobacter pylori* infection is a widespread condition that often remains asymptomatic in 90% of cases. However, this serves to be a major disadvantage as this infection can progress and result in chronic gastritis. *H. pylori* has been identified as one of the main causes of chronic gastritis. The prolonged inflammation caused by *H. pylori* can lead to significant changes in the gastric mucosa such as loss of gland and normal epithelium being replaced by collagen tissue. All this can lead to atrophic gastritis. Moreover, chronic gastritis can lead to intestinal metaplasia, a condition where the gastric epithelial cell undergoes transformation to cells that partially resemble those typically found in the small or large intestine. Both atrophic gastritis and intestinal metaplasia commonly called as chronic atrophic gastritis (CAG) are precancerous conditions, which have the potential to evolve into gastric cancer (GC) [4].

2. Prevalence and risk factors

H. pylori is a common bacterial infection that has infected 4.4 billion people worldwide, almost half of the world's population, with varying prevalences of 24–85% in different countries [1]. According to a systematic review, there is wide variation in the prevalence between regions and countries, with the highest prevalence in Africa (79%), Latin America and the Caribbean (65%), and Asia (59%). It is lowest in North America (37%) and Oceania (24.6%) [5]. It is almost ubiquitous in Southeast Asia. The prevalence varies among different countries within the same region, and it varies among different ethnic/racial groups [5]. *H. pylori* infection is chronic, and it is commonly acquired during childhood. The exact means of acquisition is unknown. It is spread from person to person through oral-oral and oral-fecal transmission. Common risk factors include age, lower socioeconomic status, certain race/ethnic groups, poor hygienic conditions such as poor sanitation, lack of access to clean water and water contamination, people with a family history of infection, certain occupations such as sheep herding, healthcare, etc. [1].

3. Pathogenesis

H. pylori colonizes the stomach's acidic environment by means of 6–8 sheathed flagella, which enable it to inhabit the gastric mucus layer. Various chemotactic factors and metals are responsible for the mobility of *H. pylori* [1]. It contains intrinsic enzymes that play an important role in colonization. First, an enzyme called urease splits urea into carbon dioxide (CO_2) and ammonia, which attenuates the acidity of the stomach environment. Second, the hydrogenase enzyme enables bacteria to use hydrogen as a source of energy. Various adhesion molecules and surface receptors help attach bacteria to gastric epithelial cells [1]. Various virulence factors, such as cytotoxin-associated gene A (Cag A) and non-Cag A factors like vacuolating cytotoxin (Vac A), duodenal ulcer promoting gene A (Dup A), outer inflammatory protein (Oip A), and gamma-glutamyl transpeptidase (GGT), induce changes in the epithelial cells, such as apoptosis, and act as proinflammatory agents [1]. Bacteria with certain virulence factors are more pathogenic than others and cause peptic ulcer disease and gastric cancer. In response to the colonization and attachment of bacteria, host cells initiate an inflammatory response mainly mediated by TH1 cells [1]. Various cytokines and interleukins are released, which are either pro-inflammatory or anti-inflammatory, leading to chronic inflammation [1]. *H. pylori* infection remains asymptomatic except in some cases where it leads to peptic ulcer, chronic gastritis, atrophic gastritis, and eventually gastric cancer [1, 6].

4. Clinical features

The clinical presentation of *H. pylori* infection is highly variable. As many as 90% of individuals infected are asymptomatic, while the other 10% can present with dyspepsia, which is defined as epigastric discomfort/pain lasting longer than one month, that may be associated with other symptoms such as nausea, early satiety, epigastric fullness, and bloating. This is often diagnosed as functional dyspepsia [6]. Symptoms correlate poorly with the severity of gastric mucosal injury seen on endoscopy, and diagnosis is often missed and not treated in time, leading to chronic gastritis or peptic ulcer disease. Due to the delay in diagnosis, peptic ulcers can present with complications such as gastrointestinal bleeding and perforation [6]. Because *H. pylori* infection remains untreated, with time chronic inflammation can lead to atrophic gastritis, which is precancerous and can progress to gastric cancer [4]. At this stage, the patient often presents with alarm symptoms such as weight loss, anemia, dysphagia, recurrent vomiting, and an epigastric/abdominal mass. Sometimes chronic gastritis can lead to other cancers, such as gastric MALT lymphoma, which presents with dyspepsia and non-specific constitutional symptoms [6]. Rarely *H. pylori* may present with extragastrointestinal manifestations such as isolated iron deficiency anemia (IDA) and idiopathic thrombocytopenic purpura (ITP) [6].

5. Diagnosis

According to the American College of Gastroenterology (ACG), *H. pylori* testing is indicated in the following cases: [6].

All patients with active PUD

- All patients with a previous history of PUD (unless it is documented that prior infection resolved) low-grade MALT lymphoma, h/o endoscopic resection of early gastric cancer
- Patients with uninvestigated dyspepsia under the age of 60 years
- Patient starting long-term NSAIDs
- Patients with unexplained iron deficiency anemia and adults with Idiopathic thrombocytopenic purpura
- In addition to it experts panel recommend a few more indications where testing is appropriate
- Patients residing in the same household as patients with proven active *H. pylori* infection.
- Patient with family history of PUD and gastric cancer

- First-generation immigrants from high-prevalence areas
- Population with a high incidence of gastric cancer

A complete history and physical examination are essential for identifying risk factors, symptoms, and signs associated with *H. pylori* infection [7]. These can include epigastric pain lasting for more than 4 weeks, or alarm symptoms like unexplained weight loss, progressive dysphagia, odynophagia, recurrent vomiting, abdominal pain, iron deficiency anemia (IDA), jaundice, gastrointestinal (GI) bleeding, and a family history of GI cancer. Following a thorough history and physical exam, appropriate diagnostic investigations should be recommended based on the assessment. There are a variety of invasive and non-invasive techniques to appropriately make the diagnosis of an *H. pylori* infection. Patients under age 55 and without alarm symptoms can be advised to go for noninvasive tests. Following are the different diagnostic investigations available in different clinical settings:

- Urea breath test (UBT): UBT requires the ingestion of urea labeled with radioactive isotopes of Carbon 13 or 14. It has a sensitivity and specificity of approximately 100%. UBT can detect active infection and can be used to confirm eradication [7].
- Stool monoclonal antigen test: This test uses monoclonal antibodies and is as accurate as UBT's when the validated test is used. This test is a cost-effective tool that can detect active infection and can be used to confirm eradication [7].
- Serological test: This test detects immunoglobulin G specific to *H. pylori* in the serum. However, it cannot distinguish between past and active infection. Serological testing can be used in cases of peptic ulcer disease (PUD) with GI bleeding or in patients with continuous NSAID use, or for mass screening [7].
- Endoscopy with biopsy: Endoscopy with biopsy can be especially useful to rule out cancer in patients with gastritis as well as to diagnose serious causes in patients aged 55 or older with one or more alarm symptoms [7]. It is also performed as a method of surveillance in patients with precancerous lesions or early gastric cancer. *H. pylori* can be detected using the rapid urease test (RUT) on biopsy specimens if the patient has not taken antibiotics for 4 weeks and proton pump inhibitors (PPIs) for 2 weeks. RUT is an accurate and cost-effective method [7]. If the above conditions are not met, *H. pylori* can be diagnosed using histology with or without RUT, culture, and polymerase chain reaction (PCR), which allows for susceptibility testing [7].

6. Treatment

All treatment guidelines agree that the best approach to the treatment of *H. pylori* is to be successful in the first attempt, thereby avoiding retreatment and reducing costs, anxiety, and further promotion of resistant strains [8]. *H. pylori*, in contrast to other bacterial gastrointestinal infections, requires a combination of antibiotics. Various factors, such as the slow growth rate of *H. pylori*, bacterial virulence, the inability of the drug to reach an appropriate level in the gastric mucus layer, and inactivation of antibiotics at low pH levels, make it difficult to eradicate with any single antibiotic [8]. Commonly used antibiotics for treatment include metronidazole, clarithromycin, amoxicillin, tetracycline, and bismuth. In some cases, third-line treatments may involve the use of ciprofloxacin, moxifloxacin, levofloxacin, furazolidone, or rifabutin [8].

H. pylori treatment requires different combinations of the antibiotics mentioned above, combined with bismuth salt or an acid-suppressive agent, as none of the above-mentioned antibiotics can work as monotherapy [8]. The rationale for adding an acid-suppressive agent, either a proton pump inhibitor PPI or an H2 receptor blocker, to the regimen is that it increases gastric pH, hence extending the half-life of antibiotics and altering the microenvironment of the bacterium [8]. Moreover, some PPIs have antimicrobial activity, which helps reduce the side effects of the given antibiotics and improves compliance [2, 8]. Bismuth compounds have been used in the treatment of peptic ulcers since the 19th century. Colloidal bismuth subcitrate, bismuth subsalicylate, and ranitidine bismuth citrate are commonly used as part of anti-*H. pylori* therapy. The mode of action of bismuth salts is complex and includes inhibition of protein synthesis, adenosine triphosphate (ATP), and cell wall, working synergistically with antibiotics and increasing the efficacy of anti-*H. pylori* therapy [8].

6.1 Standard therapy

The standard triple therapy for *H. pylori* treatment consists of amoxicillin/clarithromycin and a PPI or metronidazole/clarithromycin with a PPI given daily for 7–14 days. Studies have shown that a 14-day duration of triple therapy is much more effective and achieves a higher eradication rate compared to a 7-day therapy [7]. However, this treatment has been shown to fail 20–30% of the time due to poor compliance, prescription errors, short treatment duration, or resistance [8]. Due to increasing resistance to clarithromycin, it is recommended as first-line therapy in places/regions where resistance is lower than 15% [1]. An alternative to standard triple therapy is to combine amoxicillin, metronidazole, and clarithromycin with a PPI for 10–14 days, known as a concomitant treatment, which has better eradication rates compared to standard triple therapy [1, 7]. Adding probiotic to standard triple therapy, specifically Saccharomyces boulardii and Lactobacillus, improves eradication rates, reduces adverse effects, and improves compliance [7].

6.2 Sequential therapy

Sequential therapy consists of a five-day course of a PPI and amoxicillin twice a day, followed by a five-day course of a PPI with clarithromycin and metronidazole or tinidazole. The overall eradication rate for sequential therapy is 84%, with an eradication rate of 74% in areas where clarithromycin resistance is prevalent [7]. Sequential therapy has been shown to be superior to standard triple therapy for a 7-day duration but not superior to standard triple therapy for a 14-day duration, bismuth quadruple therapy (BQT), or non-bismuth quadruple therapy [9]. Moreover, sequential therapy has comparable compliance, incidence of side effects, and therapy interruption rates compared to standard therapy [9]. It has shown positive outcomes in both pediatric and geriatric populations, with a trial enrolling patients over 65 years of age showing better outcomes in patients treated with sequential therapy compared to the standard therapy regimen [10].

6.3 Bismuth-based quadruple therapy

Bismuth-based quadruple therapy is emerging as an alternative choice for first-line treatment in multiple studies. It includes a bismuth salt (subsalicylate or subcitrate) with metronidazole, tetracycline, and a PPI, all taken four times daily for 10–14 days. The eradication rate of a 10-day bismuth-based therapy was 90.4%, and a 14-day therapy had a rate of 97.1%, indicating that an increased duration correlated with better eradication of *H. pylori* infection [11]. This therapy is primarily used when penicillin cannot be used or when clarithromycin resistance is over 15% [12]. It is often used as salvage therapy when first-line therapy fails [6]. Longer treatment durations and consideration of metronidazole resistance are highlighted as important factors for achieving higher eradication rates [12].

6.4 Non-bismuth-based quadruple therapy

Non-bismuth-based quadruple therapy, also known as concomitant therapy, involves a combination of a PPI with amoxicillin, metronidazole, or tinidazole, and clarithromycin, given twice daily for 10–14 days. It has the highest eradication rates of about 90%, even in areas of high metronidazole and clarithromycin resistance [7]. However, the success rate of a 7-day concomitant therapy has decreased due to changes in clarithromycin resistance patterns [13].

6.5 Levofloxacin-based triple therapy

Levofloxacin-based triple therapy consists of a combination of a PPI and amoxicillin given twice daily, with levofloxacin given once daily. It can be used as salvage therapy and is better tolerated than bismuth-based quadruple therapy [7]. Levofloxacin can also be given as sequential therapy, consisting of a PPI with amoxicillin for 5–7 days, followed by a PPI with levofloxacin and nitroimidazole for 5–7 days, or as quadruple therapy, composed of levofloxacin, a PPI, nitazoxanide, and doxycycline administered for 7 or 10 days [14].

6.6 Rifabutin triple therapy

Rifabutin triple therapy has also been highlighted as effective in *H. pylori* eradication, and most guidelines recommend it as salvage therapy when first-line therapy fails [2, 6]. It consists of amoxicillin 1 g, omeprazole 40 mg, and rifabutin 50 mg for 14 days [2].

7. Salvage therapy

In case of first-line treatment failure or persistent symptoms, salvage therapy should be based on knowledge of previous antibiotics used and local resistance data [6]. Patients who experience treatment failure are either treated with second-line agents, prolonged treatment, or the addition of bismuth salts [6]. The most commonly used second-line regimen consists of a combination of tetracycline, amoxicillin/metronidazole, a PPI, and bismuth given daily for 10 days [6].

BQT or levofloxacin triple therapy is the preferred treatment option if the patient was previously treated with clarithromycin-containing first-line therapy. Clarithromycin or levofloxacin-containing treatment is considered if the patient received first-line BQT [15]. Clarithromycin triple therapy should not be considered in second-line treatment [14]. Combinations that can be considered for salvage treatment are BQT, levofloxacin triple therapy, concomitant therapy, rifabutin triple therapy, and high-dose dual therapy [14].

Due to the limited number of antibiotics that are effective against *H. pylori* and the interpatient and local differences in primary and secondary antibiotic resistance, there is no standard third-line regimen, and treatment should be based on endoscopy with bacterial culture and susceptibility testing [6].

8. Prevalence and clinical consequences of antibiotic resistance

One of the biggest challenges in *H. pylori* treatment is the growing antibiotic resistance against agents used in first-line treatment. Therefore, it is crucial to monitor the prevalence of resistance in local settings [6]. Numerous studies have shown that antibiotic resistance reduces the success rate of different anti-*H. pylori* therapies. However, the extent to which it clinically affects the outcomes depends on the different components used, the dose of each antibiotic, and the level of resistance present in *H. pylori* strains [8]. For example, studies have shown that success rates of nitroimidazole-containing PPI-based triple therapy drop from 90% in susceptible strains to 73% in resistant strains. The addition of bismuth salt to nitroimidazole-containing triple therapy increases the success rate to 92% in nitroimidazole-susceptible strains compared to 83% in resistant strains [8].

Limited studies have shown that macrolide resistance substantially reduces the efficacy of macrolide-containing *H. pylori* therapy [8]. The efficacy/success rate of adding macrolide to triple therapy may decrease from 86% in susceptible strains to 25% in resistant strains [8].

Antibiotic resistance is a growing problem worldwide, and its prevalence varies in different countries within the Asia Pacific region [15]. Data from the first-ever comprehensive systematic review and meta-analysis of primary antibiotic resistance against *H. pylori* in the past 25 years showed that the mean overall prevalence of resistance to clarithromycin was 17%, ranging from 0% in Bhutan and Myanmar to 37% in Bangladesh [15]. Clarithromycin resistance increased from 7% before 2000 to 21% in 2011–2015, according to sub-analysis of the data [15]. In the Asia Pacific region, clarithromycin resistance was higher than 15% in countries such as Bangladesh, China, India, Iran, Japan, Nepal, New Zealand, Pakistan, Saudi Arabia, Singapore, South Korea, Turkey, and Vietnam. Clarithromycin resistance was less than 15% in countries such as Bhutan, Indonesia, Laos, Malaysia, Myanmar, Russia, Taiwan, and Thailand [15]. The southeastern Asia region has the lowest risk of clarithromycin resistance [15]. Due to the growing resistance over time in the Asia Pacific region, the efficacy of clarithromycin-based triple therapy, sequential/concomitant therapy, was lower than 80% in countries with clarithromycin resistance over 20% [15].

Metronidazole resistance is common throughout the world, reflecting the frequent use of this antibiotic in medical settings [15]. The mean overall prevalence of resistance to metronidazole was 44%, ranging from 10% in Japan to 84% in Bangladesh and 88%

in Nepal [15]. Data from 2006 to 2015 showed that metronidazole resistance was higher than 40% in most countries except Japan, Myanmar, South Korea, Taiwan, and Thailand [14]. Metronidazole resistance in the Asia Pacific region was 47%, which falls between the reported rates from Europe (35%) and Latin America (50%) [15].

The mean overall prevalence of resistance to levofloxacin was 18%, ranging from 2% in Bhutan to 66% in Bangladesh [15]. Levofloxacin resistance increased from 2% before 2000 to 27% in 2011–2015, according to sub-analysis of the data [15]. Levofloxacin resistance in the Asia Pacific region was higher (21%) compared to Europe (13%) and Latin America (19%) [15].

The mean overall prevalence of resistance to amoxicillin and tetracycline was 3% and 4%, respectively, reflecting lower use of these antibiotics in medical settings [15].

These findings collectively suggest that clarithromycin-based triple therapy can be used as first-line treatment in countries where resistance is below 15% and bismuth-based quadruple therapy and non-bismuth-based quadruple therapy should be considered where clarithromycin resistance is over 15% [15].

Due to the unavailability of molecular testing or culture and susceptibility testing in most parts of the world, empiric therapy is recommended [2]. However, empiric therapy should be based on knowledge of the patient's previous antibiotic exposure, penicillin allergy, and local resistance rates. According to the ACG guideline, BQT, concomitant/non-bismuth quadruple therapy, and clarithromycin-based triple therapy are considered first-line therapy for *H. pylori* eradication [2]. Macrolide-based triple therapy is to be used when there is no previous exposure to it and in regions where local resistance is less than 15% [2].

In summary, eradication is recommended in all patients with PUD and gastric cancer. First-line therapy should have an eradication rate of more than 80%. Since pretreatment susceptibility is rarely done in primary care settings, therapy is chosen empirically based on regional bacterial resistance patterns, local recommendations, knowledge of previous antibiotic use, drug allergy, and drug availability.

9. Recent developments in *H. pylori* treatment

Due to the lack of culture and sensitivity testing and growing resistance against clarithromycin and metronidazole, bismuth quadruple therapy is considered a reliable empiric choice of treatment. A recent systematic review and meta-analysis showed that both BQT and high-dose dual therapy achieve similar eradication rates, with high-dose dual therapy having better adherence and fewer side effects. High-dose dual therapy involves using a high dose of a proton pump inhibitor (PPI) with 3 g of amoxicillin given daily for 14 days. This regimen achieves eradication rates of around 70–89% in patients with one or more prior treatment failures, and all major guidelines have recommended high-dose dual therapy [2].

Another development in *H. pylori* treatment is the approval of a new combination product containing omeprazole, rifabutin, and amoxicillin. In the ERADICATE Hp2 trial, this regimen successfully eradicated *H. pylori* in 84% of patients. The recommended treatment dose consists of 4 capsules to be taken 3 times daily. The daily dose of omeprazole is 120 mg, rifabutin is 150 mg, and amoxicillin is 3 g, which are given in equally divided capsules. The pack contains 12 identical capsules of the single combination product. In future research, the focus will be on developing narrow-spectrum agents that have specific targets, as numerous genomes of *H. pylori* have been sequenced and various newer drug therapies are under development [2].

10. Benefits of eradication therapy

Peptic ulcer disease: Eradication therapy heals most cases of PUD and greatly diminishes the risk of recurrent bleeding. A systematic review found that eradication therapy is more effective than antisecretory therapy without eradication in preventing recurrent bleeding [8, 14].

Uninvestigated dyspepsia: It is one of the indications for the diagnosis and treatment of *H. pylori* infection according to ACG guidelines. Studies have shown that the "test and treat" strategy is cost-effective and useful compared to acid-suppressive treatment in patients with uninvestigated dyspepsia. However, it is not effective in patients aged above 55 with alarm symptoms and is subject to regional *H. pylori* prevalence [14].

Functional dyspepsia or non-ulcer dyspepsia (FD): A Cochrane systematic review published in 2006 showed a small but statistically significant benefit of treating *H. pylori* infection in patients with FD, with a number needed to treat (NNT) of 14 [14].

Chronic atrophic gastritis (CAG): *H. pylori* infection is the most common cause of atrophic gastritis (AG). Multiple studies had demonstrated a strong relationship between *H. pylori* infection and the development of chronic atrophic gastritis [4]. Based on a meta-analysis, the rate ratio of AG incidence in patients with vs. without *H. pylori* infection was 5.0 (95% CI 3.1–8.30), and AG incidence was very low (<1% annually) among *H. pylori* uninfected individuals, supporting the strong relationship between *H. pylori* and AG [4]. CAG is a precancerous condition that can progress to dysplasia, and gastric cancer (GC). The rate of progression of AG to adenocarcinoma is 0.1–0.3% per year but may be higher depending on AG severity, extent, concomitant IM, and other factors The vast majority of patients with AG have evidence of current or past *H. pylori* infection [4]. Therefore, eradication of *H. pylori* is of utmost importance among anyone infected. Successful treatment and eradication of *H. pylori* can lead to the restoration of normal gastric mucosa in some patients [4]. Although not all cases show improvement, numerous studies have demonstrated a significant reduction in the risk of gastric cancer associated with *H. pylori* eradication [4].

MALT lymphoma: MALT lymphoma is now largely supplanted by marginal zone B cell lymphoma of MALT type. For patients with MALT lymphoma who have *H. pylori* infection, studies have shown that the tumor regresses in 60–93% of patients after eradication. However, the response can be inconsistent, with some patients showing a delayed response or experiencing tumor relapse within one year of treatment [14].

Early gastric cancer: Studies have shown that the incidence of metachronous gastric cancer following endoscopic resection of gastric neoplasm was reduced following eradication therapy [14].

NSAIDs: *H. pylori* is an independent risk factor for NSAID-induced ulcers and ulcer-like bleeding. Eradication of *H. pylori* before starting NSAID treatment reduces the development of ulcers and the risk of ulcer bleeding, with a 57% reduction in the incidence of peptic ulcers. The benefits are most prominent in NSAID-naive patients [14].

Asymptomatic individuals and gastric cancer: Evidence suggests that eradication reverses the gastric premalignant changes of gastric atrophy and intestinal metaplasia, although conflicting findings exist. However, studies have shown that the incidence of gastric cancer among asymptomatic individuals is reduced after eradication therapy vs. placebo or no treatment, with an NNT of 124. The estimated benefit in the population with a high risk of gastric cancer will be higher, with an estimated NNT of 15 [14].

Iron deficiency anemia (IDA): Adults with iron deficiency anemia benefit from combining iron treatment with eradication treatment, resulting in an increase in hemoglobin (Hb), serum iron, and serum ferritin levels (p-value 0.00001) [14].

Idiopathic thrombocytopenic purpura (ITP): There is limited evidence from both randomized and nonrandomized trials that there is sustained improvement in platelet count after eradication of *H. pylori* in a proportion of adults with ITP. The American Society of Hematology suggests screening for *H. pylori* infection in adults with ITP and offering eradication therapy if they test positive for an active infection [14].

11. Acid suppression with potassium-competitive acid blockers

Vonoprazan is the first and most extensively studied potassium-competitive acid blocker (P-CAB). Vonoprazan has a rapid onset of action, longer duration of action, and more profound acid suppression compared to PPIs. It is currently undergoing phase 3 clinical trials in the USA and Europe, and so far, it has yielded promising results in both dual and triple therapy [2].

12. Role of probiotics in management

Probiotics are given as an adjuvant treatment with eradication therapy as they improve eradication rates, reduce the side effects of antibiotics, and improve compliance. However, the strength of the evidence supporting their use is not strong enough because studies are either of weak quality or have a potential risk of bias. There is no strong evidence to suggest that single-strain probiotics work better than multiple-strain probiotics [1].

13. Role of *H. pylori* vaccine

Efforts to develop a vaccine against *H. pylori* have had little success over the last three decades. However, a large phase 3 clinical trial in China of an oral vaccine containing urease B has shown over 70% protection against infection. Nevertheless, the vaccine is not yet available, and more data is required before it can be widely used [1].

14. Follow-up

After treatment, it is important to assess the success or failure of the treatment. The optimal testing time depends on the choice of treatment and the test used. However, it is generally recommended to retest after four weeks of stopping antibiotics and two weeks after discontinuing PPI therapy. Various methods, both invasive and non-invasive, can be used for retesting, including the UBT, stool antigen test, and endoscopy [16]. According to the ACG, UBT or stool antigen test should be performed to confirm the eradication of *H. pylori* [16]. Endoscopy is indicated after treatment of *H. pylori* infection in two conditions: complicated PUD and gastric ulcer. The most common complications of PUD are bleeding, perforation, and obstruction/stenosis, which require either endoscopy/surgery for initial management. Non-invasive methods cannot be used in these cases because patients should be on a prolonged course of PPI, thus endoscopy is usually done to confirm eradication after treatment [16].

Gastric ulcer carries the risk of underlying malignancy, and therefore retesting with endoscopy and biopsy is necessary following eradication [16]. This not only confirms the eradication status with absolute certainty but also allows for the assessment of any underlying risk of malignancy by obtaining a biopsy from the margin of the ulcer. In cases of gastric ulcer, both before and after treatment biopsy is indicated to exclude malignancy [16]. However, in places where advanced endoscopy with new imaging techniques is available, if an ulcer appears benign with regular margins, repeat endoscopy after eradication may not be necessary [16]. Endoscopy is indicated after eradication in conditions such as for surveillance of premalignant lesions, early gastric cancer, familial gastric cancer, and gastric MALT lymphoma. The frequency of surveillance depends on the underlying conditions [16].

15. Conditions in which retesting may be considered

In cases of non-ulcer dyspepsia (functional dyspepsia), which has a poor correlation with *H. pylori*, a test-and-treat strategy is typically used. However, if symptoms persist or recur following 6–12 months of treatment, retesting is indicated. For uninvestigated dyspepsia, retesting is indicated if symptoms recur or persist after 4 weeks of treatment [16]. In most cases of chronic gastritis, successful eradication leads to the healing of gastritis and a reduced risk of developing complications [16].

Certain risk factors may warrant surveillance in patients with *H. pylori* gastritis. These risk factors include:

Presence of precancerous lesions: In some cases, *H. pylori* gastritis can progress to more severe forms of gastritis, such as atrophic gastritis or intestinal metaplasia. These conditions are considered precancerous as they increase the risk of developing gastric cancer. Surveillance endoscopy may be recommended in patients with these precancerous lesions to monitor for any signs of dysplasia or gastric cancer.

Family history of gastric cancer: Patients with a family history of gastric cancer may have a higher risk of developing the disease themselves. In such cases, surveillance endoscopy might be considered to detect any early signs of gastric cancer.

Persistent symptoms or alarm features: If a patient continues to experience persistent symptoms such as recurrent abdominal pain, bleeding, or unintended weight loss despite successful eradication of *H. pylori*, further evaluation with endoscopy may be necessary to investigate the underlying cause.

16. Recurrence

Several factors have been implicated in the recurrence of *H. pylori* infections. These factors include coming from a low socioeconomic background (low income), poor hygiene, dining out in establishments, and undergoing invasive approaches for diagnosis and treatment [17].

Author details

Malika Taufiq[1*] and Maliha Taufiq[2]

1 Mums Care Hospital, Lusaka, Zambia

2 Medical College, Aga Khan University, Karachi, Pakistan

*Address all correspondence to: drmalika76@gmail.com

References

[1] De Brito BB, Da Silva FAF, Soares AS, Pereira VA, Santos MLC, Sampaio MM, et al. Pathogenesis and clinical management of *Helicobacter pylori* gastric infection. World Journal of Gastroenterology. 2019;**25**(37):5578-5589. DOI: 10.3748/wjg.v25.i37.5578

[2] Saleem N, Howden CW. Update on the Management of *Helicobacter pylori* infection. Current Treatment Options in Gastroenterology. 2020;**18**(3):476-487. DOI: 10.1007/s11938-020-00300-3. Epub 2020 Jul 17

[3] Wang YK, Kuo FC, Liu CJ, Wu MC, Shih HY, Wang SS, et al. Diagnosis of *Helicobacter pylori* infection: Current options and developments. World Journal of Gastroenterology. 2015;**21**(40):11221-11235. DOI: 10.3748/wjg.v21.i40.11221

[4] Shah SC, Piazuelo MB, Kuipers EJ, Li D. AGA clinical practice update on the diagnosis and management of atrophic gastritis: Expert review. Gastroenterology. 2021;**161**(4):1325-1332.e7. DOI: 10.1053/j.gastro.2021.06.078. Epub 2021 Aug 26

[5] Hooi JKY, Lai WY, Ng WK, Suen MMY, Underwood FE, Tanyingoh D, et al. Global prevalence of *Helicobacter pylori* infection: Systematic review and meta-analysis. Gastroenterology. 2017;**153**(2):420-429. DOI: 10.1053/j.gastro.2017.04.022. Epub 2017 Apr 27

[6] Shatila M, Thomas AS. Current and future perspectives in the diagnosis and management of *Helicobacter pylori* infection. Journal of Clinical Medicine. 2022;**11**(17):5086. DOI: 10.3390/jcm11175086

[7] Fashner J, Gitu AC. Diagnosis and treatment of peptic ulcer disease and *H. pylori* infection. American Family Physician. 2015;**91**(4):236-242

[8] Gerrits MM, van Vliet AH, Kuipers EJ, Kusters JG. *Helicobacter pylori* and antimicrobial resistance: Molecular mechanisms and clinical implications. The Lancet Infectious Diseases. 2006;**6**(11):699-709. DOI: 10.1016/S1473-3099(06)70627-2

[9] Vaira D, Zullo A, Hassan C, Fiorini G, Vakil N. Sequential therapy for *Helicobacter pylori* eradication: The time is now! Therapeutic Advances in Gastroenterology. 2009;**2**(6):317-322. DOI: 10.1177/1756283X09343326

[10] Zullo A, Gatta L, De Francesco V, Hassan C, Ricci C, Bernabucci V, et al. High rate of *Helicobacter pylori* eradication with sequential therapy in elderly patients with peptic ulcer: A prospective controlled study. Alimentary Pharmacology & Therapeutics. 2005;**21**(12):1419-1424. DOI: 10.1111/j.1365-2036.2005.02519.x

[11] Salazar CO, Cardenas VM, Reddy RK, Dominguez DC, Snyder LK, Graham DY. Greater than 95% success with 14-day bismuth quadruple anti-*Helicobacter pylori* therapy: A pilot study in US Hispanics. Helicobacter. 2012;**17**(5):382-390

[12] Graham DY, Lee SY. How to effectively use bismuth quadruple therapy: The good, the bad, and the ugly. Gastroenterology Clinics of North America. 2015;**44**(3):537-563. DOI: 10.1016/j.gtc.2015.05.003. Epub 2015 Jun 19

[13] Huang T, Yang S, Tai W, Liang C, Kuo C, Yao C, et al. The efficacies of non-bismuth containing quadruple

therapies in the treatment of first-line anti-*Helicobacter pylori* across 4-year time interval with changing antibiotics resistance. Biomedical Journal. 2021;**44**(6):S275-S281. DOI: 10.1016/j.bj.2020.11.012

[14] Chey WD, Leontiadis GI, Howden CW, Moss SF. ACG clinical guideline: Treatment of *Helicobacter pylori* infection. American Journal of Gastroenterology. 2017;**112**(2):212-239. DOI: 10.1038/ajg.2016.563. Epub 2017 Jan 10. Erratum in: Am J Gastroenterol. 2018 Jul;113(7):1102

[15] Kuo YT, Liou JM, El-Omar EM, Wu JY, Leow AHR, Goh KL, et al. Primary antibiotic resistance in Helicobacter pylori in the Asia-Pacific region: A systematic review and meta-analysis. Lancet Gastroenterología y Hepatología. 2017;**2**(10):707-715. DOI: 10.1016/S2468-1253(17)30219-4. Epub 2017 Aug 7

[16] Kuipers EJ. When is endoscopic follow-up appropriate after *Helicobacter pylori* eradication therapy? Gastroenterology Clinics of North America. 2015;**44**(3):597-608. DOI: 10.1016/j.gtc.2015.05.006. Epub 2015 Jun 19

[17] Xue Y, Zhou LY, Lu HP, Liu JZ. Recurrence of *Helicobacter pylori* infection: Incidence and influential factors. Chinese Medical Journal. 2019;**132**(7):765-771. DOI: 10.1097/CM9.0000000000000146

Section 4

Medical Health Care in Tertiary Level Hospitals

Chapter 7

Bowel Preparation before Elective Colorectal Surgery: Its Current Role

Navin Kumar, Aakansha Giri Goswami, Dhiraj Mallik, Sudhir Kumar Singh, Farhanul Huda and Somprakas Basu

Abstract

Bowel preparation for elective colorectal surgery has been performed for decades with the assumption to decrease infectious complications and anastomotic leaks. Nevertheless, the scientific basis of the same is still debatable. Various methods of bowel preparation are mechanical bowel preparation (MBP) with or without prophylactic oral antibiotics (POA), preoperative POA alone without MBP, and preoperative enema alone without MBP and POA. However, there is no consensus on the optimal type of bowel preparation. The available agents for MBP are polyethylene glycol (PEG) and sodium phosphate (NaP) or picosulphate. The most common prophylactic oral antibiotic regimen used in preoperative bowel preparation is Neomycin and Metronidazole a day before surgery, although the microbiological basis of this is unverified. Most studies around the beginning of this century indicate inadequate evidence for using MBP for colorectal surgery to suggest harm caused by the process and accordingly advise against it. However, several retrospective studies and meta-analyses, which were done after 2014, arguably demonstrate that preoperative MBP and POA reduce the postoperative surgical site infection rate. However, as per the current evidence, it can be suggested that MBP and preoperative POA can be safely included in the preoperative preparation of elective colorectal surgery.

Keywords: bowel preparation, colorectal surgery, mechanical bowel preparation, laparoscopic colorectal surgery, antibiotics, rectal surgery

1. Introduction

Bowel preparation refers to the mechanical cleansing of the bowel through the oral, rectal route, or a combined route. It has been in use for many decades as a part of preoperative preparation before elective colorectal surgery. However, the scientific basis of this practice is still debatable [1]. The infectious complication and anastomotic leak (2.7–20%) are the significant issues with colorectal surgery. These lead to increased morbidity in terms of postoperative ileus (10–30%), surgical site infection (6.5–20%), re-admission rate (8.1–11.8%), and an increase in the length of hospital stay (LOS) [1–7]. Colonic bacterial flora is one of the major causes of infectious complications in colorectal surgery, but the effective way to reduce the bacterial load is still debatable [8]. Preoperative bowel preparation is one of the techniques frequently studied to reduce these colonic bacterial florae. It is not easy to indicate when mechanical bowel preparation (MBP) was first used in colorectal surgery and is still the subject of debate.

Nevertheless, it is believed that preoperative mechanical bowel preparation (MBP) removes stool content and associated bacterial load, thereby reducing surgical site infection (SSI). The other benefit of MBP is easier bowel manipulation during surgery [9]. Subsequently, nonabsorbable antibiotics were added to reduce the bacterial load further. Since 1970, MBP plus poorly absorbed prophylactic oral antibiotics (POA) and intravenous antibiotics effective against intestinal microorganisms were accepted before elective colorectal surgery [10]. However, the effect of antibiotics is believed to last beyond the surgical intervention and can influence the structure and function of the gut microbiome [11]. The human intestine possesses millions of microbial genes, known as microbiome [12]. These microbiomes are highly specific, which is the reason for the conflicting data of MBP or the combination of MBP with POA [13]. Multiple clinical trials have been conducted to determine the best strategy for bowel preparation, but their results are controversial [14–16]. Since 1980, the evidence of Enhanced Recovery After Surgery (ERAS) and the successful outcome of emergency colorectal surgery has led to the belief that MBP can be omitted.

Many RCTs have failed to demonstrate any protective benefit of isolated MBP against infective complications or anastomotic leaks. On the contrary, the patients exhibited a paradoxical increase in postoperative ileus. Data from the late twentieth century studies suggest that the elimination of MBP does not increase morbidity. This gradually led to a trend of avoiding MBP routinely. Nevertheless, most of these studies have not combined the POA with MBP. Preoperative POA use has also decreased as surgeons started following ERAS. But the use of POA has not disappeared completely [17–20]. There is a resurgence of bowel preparation because of the high risk of surgical site infection after colorectal surgery. Since 2013, clinical guidelines have been changing, and a combination of MBP and POA is now recommended [21–23]. A number of retrospective studies and meta-analyses have been done after 2014, which have shown that preoperative MBP and POA following colorectal surgery reduce postoperative surgical site infection [24–28].

There are various methods of bowel preparation before elective colorectal surgery. These include MBP alone without a preoperative POA, MBP with preoperative POA, preoperative POA alone without MBP, and preoperative enema alone without MBP and POA. However, there is no consensus on the optimal type of bowel preparation, and it generally depends on the treating surgeon's preference and the patient's prognosis [29]. However, most surgeons prefer preoperative POA with MBP in elective colorectal surgery.

1.1 MBP alone

Before elective colorectal surgery, MBP was a standard method of care for over a century. The earliest mention in the literature about the practice of bowel decontamination was published in British Medical Journal in November 1899 by Burney Yeo in his article "a discussion of intestinal antiseptics" [30]. It has been performed since 1930 without any clear evidence of a reduction in complication [31]. There is a long history of research on preoperative MBP in colorectal surgery [32]. The most debated aspect of bowel preparation is its role in reducing surgical morbidity, such as surgical site infection (SSI) [29]. The SSI rate is highest in colorectal surgery, which varies between 5.4% and 23.2%, with a mean of 11.4% [33]. However, the evidence does not show any benefit of MBP in reducing the mucosa-associated bacterial load in the colon. Preoperative preparation before elective colorectal surgery was shifted to outpatient care, and the mortality rate continued to decrease. Surgeons started questioning the need for the MBP, and many centers appeared to confirm the abandonment of MBP [34]. One multicenter randomized control trial (RCT) published by Contant et al. with 1345 patients did not demonstrate any significant difference in anastomotic leak rates between patients who received MBP (n = 670) and those who did not (n = 684) [35]. In 2007, Jung et al. published another retrospective study of 1343 cases that reported similar results and suggested the omission of MBP before colorectal surgery [36]. Bucher et al. demonstrated significant adverse effects associated with MBP, such as loss of superficial mucus and infiltration of polymorphonuclear cells and lymphocytes suggesting inflammatory changes in the mucosa [37]. Several case reports demonstrated adverse side effects of MBP such as seizures and electrolyte imbalance such as hyponatremia, hypernatremia, hypocalcemia, and hyperphosphatemia [38–41]. The available agents for MBP are polyethylene glycol (PEG), sodium phosphate (NaP), and picosulphate. They have unpleasant side effects as well as the process is time-consuming. The preparation of sodium phosphate is palatable and made in 300 ml of water [42]. It principally acts as a purgative. Although it is better tolerated by the patients but is associated with fluid and electrolyte imbalance. It should not be given in patients with congestive cardiac failure, cirrhosis, or chronic kidney disease [43]. Full MBP in most RCT is done with an osmotic agent such as PEG with an electrolyte solution. The PEG–electrolyte solution is prepared in 2 liters (L) of water. The patient drinks 2 L of PEG–electrolyte solution and 1 L of clear fluid. PEG electrolyte solution minimizes fluid and electrolyte imbalance [44]. The outcome of agents such as sodium phosphate (NaP) or picosulphate in bowel preparation has not been studied as much as has been done with PEG. A clinical trial by Itani et al. in 2007 compared PEG with sodium phosphate and concluded that sodium phosphate is superior to PEG in bowel preparation [45]. Sodium phosphate (NaP) can be used as an enema or an oral preparation, but PEG is used as oral preparation only. The unclear benefit of MBP is a reduction in bacterial load within the bowel as it removes solid fecal content, makes easier manipulation of the bowel during surgery, and helps in performing intraoperative colonoscopy if needed. A number of RCTs [15, 16, 46–54], meta-analyses [55–63], and one Cochrane review [63] on MBP have been published but none of these have conclusively recommended any significant benefit of MBP alone in elective colorectal surgery. MBP has possible disadvantages, such as patient discomfort in the form of nausea, vomiting, abdominal distension, insomnia, and weakness. Other significant complications include fluid and electrolyte imbalance and alteration of gut microbiota and colonic mucus layer, which has been shown to cause increased bacterial translocation [37, 64]. However, the addition of nonabsorbable oral antibiotics with MBP decreases the SSI rates by approximately 40% when compared with that of MBP alone [25, 65, 66]. Many research studies have also evaluated bowel preparation with rectal enema alone without MBP and POA, and have observed a similar rate of wound infection and anastomotic dehiscence. However, bowel preparation with rectal enema alone without MBP and POA is not recommended (weak recommendation based on moderate-quality evidence, 2B) [67]. Preoperative MBP alone, without POA, is also not recommended for patients undergoing elective colorectal surgery (Grade of recommendation: strong recommendation based on high-quality evidence, 1A) [68].

1.2 MBP plus preoperative prophylactic oral antibiotics

Another aspect of bowel preparation is adding preoperative prophylactic oral antibiotics (POA) with MBP. Bowel preparation before colorectal surgery with POA was first proposed by Poth et al. in 1942 [69]. Whereas the combination of POA with MBP before elective colorectal surgery was introduced by Nichols et al. in 1971 [70]. In their landmark prospective randomized control trial comparing MBP with or without preoperative nonabsorbable oral antibiotics, Nichols et al. concluded a marked decrease in SSI with the use of a combination of MBP and POA [8, 70]. In their RCT, they used neomycin and erythromycin base and MBP. Interestingly, other studies have failed to demonstrate any significant protective benefit of this regimen against postoperative complications. Nichols et al., from their study, concluded that MBP did not decrease the microbial burden; rather, it facilitated the effect of oral antibiotics to decrease the mucosal concentration of bacteria [8, 70]. In 1980, most American and Canadian surgeons started using oral and parenteral antibiotic prophylaxis and MBP [71]. Later Smith MB et al., in 1990, highlighted the importance of oral antibiotics over intravenous antibiotics [72]. In 2002, Lewis conducted a prospective trial comparing parenteral antibiotics alone with a combination of parenteral and oral antibiotics. However, MBP was done in both these groups. He reported a lower incidence of SSI in the oral and parenteral antibiotic group [73]. In 2010, Markell et al., in their study, showed that only 39% of surgeons are using a POA, which was a substantial decrease in oral antibiotics use when compared to 1990 [74]. In the year 2015, combination of POA with MBP in elective colorectal surgery was reintroduced, but it became widespread in 2016 [75]. It is presumed that a combination of these two will give a synergistic effect. Nonabsorbable oral antibiotics, when combined with MBP, further reduce the intraluminal bacterial load and SSI rates [76]. However, the choice of antibiotics for this purpose is not clear. Different clinical trials have used different antibiotics, but these did not conclude which is better. Our knowledge has not moved beyond the existing formulation regimens for bowel preparation to advance our understanding of the pathogenesis of SSI and anastomotic leak. Overall perception indicates that antibiotics with both aerobic and anaerobic cover should be chosen [77]. Unfortunately, antibiotics used for bowel preparation have not changed in decades despite recognizing antibiotic resistance in surgical patients [78, 79]. Kirby et al., in their article, described the need for recalibration of antibiotics after reports from Leeds, United Kingdom, suggesting resistant Enterobacteriaceae responsible for SSI [80]. A randomized control trial by Clarke et al. demonstrated the role and efficacy of oral antibiotics in reducing SSI in elective colorectal surgery [81]. Many studies to date have demonstrated that oral nonabsorbable antibiotics before elective colorectal surgery prevent anastomotic leak more effectively than intravenous antibiotics alone [32]. The most common prophylactic oral antibiotic regimen used in these studies for preoperative bowel preparation is Neomycin (1 g) and Metronidazole (1 g) two times a day before surgery. However, the microbiological basis of this is unverified [82]. Only a few randomized clinical trials are in the literature on POA alone without MBP and POA with MBP. A recent meta-analysis conducted in 2018, which included two RCTs (n = 709) and two cohort studies (n = 22,774), did not find any difference in the overall incidence of SSI between the groups or even when RCTs and cohort studies were analyzed separately [83]. However, there is little level 1 evidence for POA alone without MBP [13], and therefore, preoperative POA without MBP is not recommended (Grade of recommendation: weak recommendation based on low-quality evidence, 2C) [29]. There is also no consensus on the optimal type of bowel preparation. Nichols et al. used the combination of oral Neomycin (1 g) and Erythromycin (1 g) dosages at 1:00 pm, 2:00 pm, and at 11:00 pm (total 6 g) a day before surgery along with MBP. They could reduce the fecal aerobic and anaerobic flora [84]. Neomycin and Erythromycin combination has been used for decades without any evidence of major side effects and many centers use a full MBP using PEG with electrolyte solution and two doses of oral Neomycin (1 g) and Metronidazole (1 g). Kim et al., in 2014, compared MBP with or without POA and found a significantly lower risk of surgical site infection (SSI) and Clostridium difficile colitis when both were used in combination. Michigan Surgical Quality Collaboration (MSQC) recommends full MBP and POA before colorectal surgery unless there is a contraindication for the same [85]. In 2015, Scarborough et al. compared the POA alone versus POA combined MBP, and their result supports the routine utilization of MBP with POA [17]. However, their POA alone group was comparatively smaller in size than the combined MBP and POA [17]. ERAS society also recommends the combination of preoperative MBP and POA before elective colorectal surgery [28]. Many centers use POA alone before elective colorectal surgery. Their results of using POA have been assessed in two large retrospective studies conducted by the American College of Surgeons National Surgical Quality Improvement Program (NSQIP) on more than 30,000 patients and one large prospective meta-analyses on 69,000 patients. These have shown almost comparable or lower SSI rates among patients who received MBP plus POA versus those who received MBP alone [27, 83, 86]. Preoperative MBP and preoperative POA in elective colorectal surgery are recommended (strong moderate-quality evidence, 1B) [75, 87–90]. Currently, the practice can be summed up as: the MBP can be started two days before surgery and must be completed one day before surgery by 15:00 hours. The patient takes 1 g of Neomycin and 1 g of Metronidazole orally after completion of MBP at 15:00 and 23:00 hours. One hour before surgery, the patient should also receive perioperative intravenous antibiotics (Cefuroxime 1.5 g and Metronidazole 500 mg). The dose of intravenous antibiotics can be repeated if the duration of surgery is more than 3 hours [44].

1.3 MBP in elective rectal surgery

Data on MBP in patients with rectal surgery are not sufficient. Traditionally rectal washouts were done. The issues related to rectal surgery are different from those of colonic surgery. In low colorectal or coloanal anastomosis (anastomosis within 6 cm from the anal verge), a protective ostomy is often made because of the higher risk of anastomotic leak. A meta-analysis conducted on 28 RCTs and 12 cohort studies with 69,517 patients concluded that a combination of POA with MBP was associated with a significant reduction of SSI ($RR = 0.51$, $p < 0.00001$), anastomotic leak ($RR = 0.62$, $p < 0.00001$), 30 days mortality ($RR = 0.58$, $p < 0.0001$), overall morbidity ($RR = 0.67$, $p < 0.00001$), and postoperative ileus ($RR = 0.72$, $p = 0.04$) [83]. Anastomotic leak after rectal surgery is higher than that in colonic surgery [91]. Bretagnol et al. conducted a study on the role of MBP in rectal surgery, and they reported a higher infectious morbidity rate in the patient without MBP [92]. In contrast, Mahajna et al. reported that MBP causes liquid bowel contents, which lead to peritoneal spillage three times more frequently than when semisolid stool is present [93]. Results are not uniform regarding the use of oral antibiotics before rectal surgery, and very few studies have been done exclusively on rectal cancer patients [94]. Zmora et al. reported that some form of bowel preparation, such as rectal enema, is required before rectal surgery [14]. Bowel preparation with rectal enema is less invasive and well-tolerated and has not been associated with increased infectious morbidity [95]. However, more multicenter trials are required to gather evidence for MBP before rectal surgery.

1.4 MBP in laparoscopic surgery

There is a rise in laparoscopic resection for colon cancer. The laparoscopic technique has brought a significant decrease in SSI [96]. However, data on MBP in laparoscopic surgery are not sufficient. Many studies have not confirmed the effectiveness of preoperative MBP before laparoscopic surgery. However, proponents of MBP still recommend MBP before laparoscopic surgery for easier manipulation of the bowel and intracorporeal stapling, and reduction of fecal contamination in case of spillage during bowel resection [97–99]. In a retrospective review, Zmora et al. compared the outcomes of 68 laparoscopic colectomies with MBP and 132 without MBP. They did not find any benefit in the complication rates in the MBP group [100]. Chan et al. also reported a comparable 4.1% and 3.8% wound infection rate, an anastomotic leak at 1% and 0.6% in the no-MBP and MBP groups, respectively [101]. However, using MBP might improve the operative space due to improved view resulting from decreased colonic distension following MBP [102]. The RCT conducted by Won et al. reported a better surgical view in patients with MBP undergoing laparoscopic colorectal surgery [103]. However, this benefit may not be available in the presence of obstructing tumor that causes a decrease in operative space because of the distension of the proximal bowel [103]. Overall, MBP is widely preferred before laparoscopic colorectal surgery, but the best option is better left to the individual surgeon's preference [104–106].

1.5 Using microbiome science to develop bowel preparation

Bowel preparation relies on the traditional paradigm [107, 108]. Still, there is a lack of recognition of the importance of normal microbiota in suppressing colonization resistance and promoting intestinal healing. The microbiota includes bacteria, viruses, fungi, and protozoans, which live symbiotically with humans. Gut microbiota (GM) are of two types. According to their location, they are named mucosal-associated microbiota (MAM) and luminal microbiota (LM). Bacteroidetes and Proteobacteria are representative of MAM, whereas Firmicutes and Actinobacteria are representative of the LM [109]. MAM stimulates the mucus secretion in the gut. It also produces short-chain fatty acids, acetate, butyrate, and propionate. These are the mediators of the host immune system. The LM, mainly Firmicutes, produces butyrate, which enhances intestinal barrier function and has anti-inflammatory and anticancer activity [110]. Studies lack how normal microbiota are reintroduced after surgery and provide health-promoting effects [111]. In the era of laparoscopic surgery, oral antibiotics may be less critical as the microbiota are minimally disturbed [94]. The intestinal decontamination, as complete as possible, should be the goal of adequate bowel preparation [112]. In current practice, by doing broad-based bowel preparation, decontamination of diverse GM happens. Diverse GM suppresses the development of potential harmful pathobionts and promotes intestinal healing. The next generation of bowel preparation using microbial metagenomics focuses on selective gut decontamination. Gentle bowel cleansing can begin with nutritional supplements and non-microbicidal anti-virulence agents. Here the nutritional supplement includes the nutrients known to suppress bacterial virulence without affecting their growth. Hence the normal GM proliferates but the virulence of pathogenic microbiota is suppressed [113]. Therefore, a balanced solution containing both nutrients and anti-virulence agents will be the next generation and more scientifically validated approach for bowel preparation before colorectal surgery that allows for targeted cleansing while preserving the vital function of the normal microbiota. However, evidence favored the MBP with POA before elective colorectal surgery. Now the time has come to allow the next-generation microbial science technology to recalibrate the traditional bowel preparation.

1.6 Bowel preparation and surgical recovery

The surgical recovery mainly focuses on the protective benefit of bowel preparation against SSI and anastomotic leak (AL), which in turn leads to increased intra-abdominal collections, reoperation rate, length of hospital stays (LOS), and 30 days' morbidity. Following colorectal surgery, about 20% of patients may suffer from SSI [114]. SSIs are associated with increased morbidity and LOS and delayed recovery. A number of high-quality studies report a reduction in SSI rates after MBP and POA [8, 70, 76, 115]. Klinger et al. analyzed subjects from the American College of Surgeons–National Surgical Quality Improvement Program (ACS-NSQIP) database and observed its protective benefit against SSI and AL rates [4, 17]. ACS-NSQIP data analysis also demonstrated a significant reduction in the readmission rate and LOS in a patient with MBP plus POA [28]. Interestingly, also it has been observed that AL following elective surgery for colorectal cancer adversely affects overall survival. It is probably because of increased local cancer recurrence as well as delays in starting the chemotherapy. Although the risk of AL is 2.2 times higher with only MBP, it decreases with the addition of POA [116], probably because the addition of POA reduces bowel bacterial colonization, which might lead to a decrease in infectious complications. Similar observations on recovery from laparoscopic colorectal surgery indicate that the LOS, complication rate, and reoperation rate decrease after the use of MBP and POA.

The protocol of enhanced recovery after surgery (ERAS) is established on the principle of reduction in surgically induced physiological and metabolic stress. The benefit of MBP plus POA can be a pillar in the ERAS pathway. ERAS society also recommends using preoperative MBP plus POA before elective colorectal surgery [28] because it reduces postoperative ileus [117], non-SSI-related complications [76], the LOS, and hospital readmission rates [118]. The ACS-NSQIP data indicate a reduction in 30-day mortality with MBP plus POA than not having bowel preparation at all, which is likely due to an overall decrease in septic complications [76]. These data suggest that bowel preparation (MBP plus POA) has a significant advantage on surgical recovery by reducing the SSIs, anastomotic leak, postoperative ileus, reoperation, and readmission rate as well as LOS and 30-day mortality.

2. Conclusion

MBP has no apparent benefit in reducing SSI when used alone. Current evidence suggests that SSI reduction occurs better when MBP is combined with POA. There is a possibility that the observed decrease in SSI might be due to the use of POA alone rather than the combination of MBP with POA. Emerging research on the microbiome will guide more specific bowel preparation regimens for the individual case. To date, the combination of preoperative MBP plus POA in elective colorectal surgery is recommended.

Funding

Nil.

Conflict of interest

The authors declare no conflict of interest.

Author details

Navin Kumar, Aakansha Giri Goswami, Dhiraj Mallik, Sudhir Kumar Singh, Farhanul Huda and Somprakas Basu*
Department of General Surgery, All India Institute of Medical Sciences, Rishikesh, India

*Address all correspondence to: somprakas.surg@aiimsrishikesh.edu.in

References

[1] Basu S, Shukla VK. Mechanical bowel preparation: Are we ready for a paradigm shift? Digestive Surgery. 2008;**25**(5):325-327

[2] Sciuto A, Merola G, De Palma GD, et al. Predictive factors for anastomotic leakage after laparoscopic colorectal surgery. World Journal of Gastroenterology. 2018;**24**(21):2247-2260

[3] Chen M, Song X, Chen LZ, et al. Comparing mechanical bowel preparation with both oral and systemic antibiotics versus mechanical bowel preparation and systemic antibiotics alone for the prevention of surgical site infection after elective colorectal surgery: A meta-analysis of randomize. Diseases of the Colon and Rectum. 2016;**59**(1):70-78

[4] Klinger AL, Green H, Monlezun DJ, et al. The role of bowel preparation in colorectal surgery: Results of the 2012-2015 ACS-NSQIP data. Annals of Surgery. 2019;**269**(4):671-677

[5] Damen N, Spilsbury K, Levitt M, et al. Anastomotic leaks in colorectal surgery. ANZ Journal of Surgery. 2014;**84**(10):763-768

[6] Toneva GD, Deierhoi RJ, Morris M, et al. Oral antibiotic bowel preparation reduces length of stay and readmissions after colorectal surgery. Journal of the American College of Surgeons. 2013;**216**(4):756-762

[7] Venara A, Neunlist M, Slim K, et al. Postoperative ileus: Pathophysiology, incidence, and prevention. Journal of Visceral Surgery. 2016;**153**(6):439-446

[8] Nichols RL, Choe EU, Weldon CB. Mechanical and antibacterial bowel preparation in colon and rectal surgery. Chemotherapy. 2005;**51**(suppl. 1): 115-121

[9] Diakosavvas M, Thomakos N, Psarris A, Fasoulakis Z, Theodora M, Haidopoulos D, et al. Preoperative bowel preparation in minimally invasive and vaginal gynecologic surgery. Scientific World-Journal. 2020;**2020**:8546037

[10] Fry DE. The prevention of surgical site infection in elective colon surgery. Scientifica (Cairo). 2013;**2013**:896297

[11] Dethlefsen L, Relman DA. Incomplete recovery and individualized responses of the human distal gut microbiotato repeated antibiotic perturbation. Proceedings of the National Academy of Sciences USA. 2011;**108**(Suppl. 1):4554-4561

[12] Kinross JM, Darzi AW, Nicholson JK. Gut microbiome–host interactions in health and disease. Genome Medicine. 2011;**3**:14

[13] Duff SE, Battersby CLF, Davies RJ, Hancock L, Pipe J, Buczacki S, et al. The use of oral antibiotics and mechanical bowel preparation in elective colorectal resection for the reduction of surgical site infection. Colorectal Disease. 2020;**22**(4):364-372

[14] Zmora O, Mahajna A, Bar-Zakai B, et al. Colon and rectal surgery without mechanical bowel preparation: A randomized prospective trial. Annals of Surgery. 2003;**237**:363-367

[15] Ram E, Sherman Y, Weil R, et al. Is mechanical bowel preparation mandatory for elective colon surgery? A prospective randomized study. Archives of Surgery. 2005;**140**:285-288

[16] Miettinen RP, Laitinen ST, Mäkelä JT, Pääkkönen ME. Bowel preparation with oral polyethylene glycol electrolyte solution vs no preparation in elective open colorectal surgery: Prospective, randomized study. Diseases of the Colon and Rectum. 2000;**43**(5):669-675

[17] Scarborough JE, Mantyh CR, Sun Z, Migaly J. Combined mechanical and oral antibiotic bowel preparation reduces incisional surgical site infection and anastomotic leak rates after elective colorectal resection: An analysis of colectomy-targeted ACS NSQIP. Annals of Surgery. 2015;**262**:331-337

[18] Platell C, Hall J. What is the role of mechanical bowel preparation in patients undergoing colorectal surgery? Diseases of the Colon and Rectum. 1998;**41**:875-883

[19] Lewis J, Kinross J. Mechanical bowel preparation for elective colorectal surgery. Techniques in Coloproctology. 2019;**23**:783-785

[20] Slim K, Vicaut E, Panis Y, Chipponi J. Meta-analysis of randomized clinical trials of colorectal surgery with or without mechanical bowel preparation. The British Journal of Surgery. 2004;**91**:1125-1130

[21] Carmichael JC, Keller DS, Baldini G, Bordeianou L, Weiss E, Lee L, et al. Clinical practice guidelines for enhanced recovery after colon and rectal surgery from the American Society of Colon and Rectal Surgeons and Society of American Gastrointestinal and Endoscopic Surgeons. Diseases of the Colon and Rectum. 2017;**60**:761-784

[22] Allegranzi B, Bischoff P, de Jonge S, Kubilay NZ, Zayed B, Gomes SM, et al. New WHO recommendations on preoperative measures for surgical site infection prevention: An evidence-based global perspective. The Lancet Infectious Diseases. 2016;**16**:e276-e287

[23] Bratzler DW, Dellinger EP, Olsen KM, Perl TM, Auwaerter PG, Bolon MK, et al. Clinical practice guidelines for antimicrobial prophylaxis in surgery. Surgical Infections. 2013;**14**:73-156

[24] Nelson RL, Gladman E, Barbateskovic M. Antimicrobial prophylaxis for colorectal surgery. Cochrane Database of Systematic Reviews. May 9, 2014;**2014**(5):CD001181

[25] Chen M, Song X, Chen LZ, Lin ZD, Zhang XL. Comparing mechanical bowel preparation with both oral and systemic antibiotics versus mechanical bowel preparation and systemic antibiotics alone for the prevention of surgical site infection after elective colorectal surgery: A meta-analysis of randomized controlled clinical trials. Diseases of the Colon and Rectum. 2016;**59**:70-78

[26] Vo E, Massarweh NN, Chai CY, et al. Association of the addition of oral antibiotics to mechanical bowel preparation for left colon and rectal cancer resections with reduction of surgical site infections. JAMA Surgery. 2018;**153**(2):114-121

[27] Koller SE, Bauer KW, Egleston BL, et al. Comparative effectiveness and risks of bowel preparation before elective colorectal surgery. Annals of Surgery. 2018;**267**(4):734-742

[28] Morris MS, Graham LA, Chu DI, et al. Oral antibiotic bowel preparation significantly reduces surgical site infection rates and readmission rates in elective colorectal surgery. Annals of Surgery. 2015;**261**(6):1034-1040

[29] Migaly J, Bafford AC, Francone TD, Gaertner WB, Eskicioglu C, Bordeianou L, et al. The

American Society of Colon and Rectal Surgeons clinical practice guidelines for the use of bowel preparation in elective colon and Rectal surgery. Diseases of the Colon and Rectum. Lippincott Williams and Wilkins. 2019;**62**:3-8

[30] Yeo B, Harley V, Goodbody F, et al. A discussion on intestinal antiseptics. British Medical Journal. 1899;**2**:1250-1257

[31] Fry DE. Antimicrobial bowel preparation for elective colon surgery. Surgical Infections. 2016;**17**:269-274

[32] Fry DE. Colon preparation and surgical site infection. American Journal of Surgery. 2011;**202**:225-232

[33] Young H, Knepper B, Moore EE, Johnson JL, Mehler P, Price CS. Surgical site infection after colon surgery: National Health-care Safety Network risk factors and modeled rates com-pared with published risk factors and rates. Journal of the American College of Surgeons. 2012;**214**:852-859

[34] Zmora O, Mahajina A, Bar-Zakai B, et al. Colon and rectal surgery without mechanical bowel preparation. Techniques in Coloproctology. 2004;**237**:363-367

[35] Contant CM, Hop WC, van't Sant HP, Oostvogel HJ, Smeets HJ, Stassen LP, et al. Mechanical bowel preparation for elective colorectal surgery: A multicentre randomised trial. Lancet. 2007;**370**:2112-2117

[36] Jung B, Påhlman L, Nyström PO, Nilsson E. Mechanical bowel preparation study group. Multi Centre randomized clinical trial of mechanical bowel preparation in elective colonic resection. The British Journal of Surgery. 2007;**94**:689-695

[37] Bucher P, Gervaz P, Egger JF, Soravia C, Morel P. Morphologic alterations associated with mechanical bowel preparation before elective colorectal surgery: A randomized trial. Diseases of the Colon and Rectum. 2006;**49**:109-112

[38] Ayus JC, Levine R, Arieff AI. Fatal dysnatraemia caused by elective colonoscopy. BMJ. 2003;**326**:382-384

[39] Hookey LC, Depew WT, Vanner S. The safety profile of oral sodium phosphate for colonic clean sing before colonoscopy in adults. Gastrointestinal Endoscopy. 2002;**56**:895-902

[40] Mackey AC, Shaffer D, Prizont R. Seizure associated with the use of visicol for colonoscopy. The New England Journal of Medicine. 2002;**346**:2095 author reply 2095

[41] Hayakawa Y, Tanaka Y, Funahashi H, et al. Hyperphosphatemia accelerates parathyroid cell proliferation and parathyroid hormone secretion in severe secondary parathyroid hyperplasia. Endocrine Journal. 1999;**46**:681-686

[42] Hsu CW, Imperiale TF. Meta-analysis and cost comparison of polyethylene glycol lavage versus sodium phosphate for colonoscopy preparation. Gastrointestinal Endoscopy. 1998;**48**:276-282

[43] Connor A, Tolan D, Hughes S, et al. Consensus guidelines for the safe prescription and administration of oral bowel-cleansing agents. Gut. 2012;**61**:1525-1532

[44] Koskenvuo L, Lunkka P, Varpe P, Hyöty M, Satokari R, Haapamäki C, et al. Mechanical bowel preparation and oral antibiotics versus mechanical bowel preparation only prior rectal surgery (MOBILE2): A multicentre, double-blinded, randomised controlled

trial—Study protocol. BMJ Open. 2021;**11**:e051269

[45] Itani KM, Wilson SE, Awad SS, Jensen EH, Finn TS, Abramson MA. Polyethylene glycol versus sodium phosphate mechanical bowel preparation in elective colorectal surgery. American Journal of Surgery. 2007;**193**:190-194

[46] Bhat AH, Parray FQ, Chowdri NA, et al. Mechanical bowel preparation versus no preparation in elective colorectal surgery: A prospective randomized study. International Journal of Surgery Open. 2016;**2**:26-30

[47] Fa-Si-Oen P, Roumen R, Buitenweg J, et al. Mechanical bowel preparation or not? Outcome of a multicenter, randomized trial in elective open colon surgery. Diseases of the Colon and Rectum. 2005;**48**:1509-1516

[48] Ali M. Randomized prospective clinical trial of NO preparation versus mechanical bowel preparation before elective colorectal surgery. Medicine Channel. 2007;**13**:32-35

[49] Bertani E, Chiappa A, Biffi R, et al. Comparison of oral polyethylene glycol plus a large volume glycerine enema with a large volume glycerine enema alone in patients undergoing colorectal surgery for malignancy: A randomized clinical trial. Colorectal Disease. 2011;**13**:e327-e334

[50] Bhattacharjee PK, Chakraborty S. An open- label prospective randomized controlled trial of mechanical bowel preparation vs nonmechanical bowel preparation in elective colorectal surgery: Personal experience. The Indian Journal of Surgery. 2015;**77**:1233-1236

[51] Bucher P, Gervaz P, Soravia C, et al. Randomized clinical trial of mechanical bowel preparation versus no preparation before elective left- sided colorectal surgery. The British Journal of Surgery. 2005;**92**:409-414

[52] Pena-Soria MJ, Mayol JM, Anula R, et al. Single- blinded randomized trial of mechanical bowel preparation for colon surgery with primary intraperitoneal anastomosis. Journal of Gastrointestinal Surgery. 2008;**12**:2103-2109

[53] Saha AK, Chowdhury F, Jha AK, et al. Mechanical bowel preparation versus no preparation before colorectal surgery: A randomized prospective trial in a tertiary care institute. Journal of Natural Science, Biology, and Medicine. 2014;**5**:421-424

[54] Sasaki J, Matsumoto S, Kan H, et al. Objective assessment of postoperative gastrointestinal motility in elective colonic resection using a radiopaque marker provides an evidence for the abandonment of preoperative mechanical bowel preparation. Journal of Nippon Medical School. 2012;**79**:259-266

[55] Bucher P, Mermillod B, Gervaz P, et al. Mechanical bowel preparation for elective colorectal surgery: A meta- analysis. Archives of Surgery. 2004;**139**:1359-1364

[56] Courtney DE, Kelly ME, Burke JP, et al. Postoperative outcomes following mechanical bowel preparation before proctectomy: A meta- analysis. Colorectal Disease. 2015;**17**:862-869

[57] Dahabreh IJ, Steele DW, Shah N, et al. Oral mechanical bowel preparation for colorectal surgery: Systematic review and meta- analysis. Diseases of the Colon and Rectum. 2015;**58**:698-707

[58] Pineda CE, Shelton AA, Hernandez-Boussard T, et al. Mechanical bowel preparation in intestinal surgery: A meta- analysis and review of the

literature. Journal of Gastrointestinal Surgery. 2008;**12**:2037-2044

[59] Rollins KE, Javanmard-Emamghissi H, Lobo DN. Impact of mechanical bowel preparation in elective colorectal surgery: A meta- analysis. World Journal of Gastroenterology. 2018;**24**:519-536

[60] Slim K, Vicaut E, Launay-Savary M-V, et al. Updated systematic review and meta- analysis of randomized clinical trials on the role of mechanical bowel preparation before colorectal surgery. Annals of Surgery. 2009;**249**:203-209

[61] Wille Jorgensen P, Guenaga KF, Matos D, et al. Pre- operative mechanical bowel cleansing or not? An updated meta- analysis. Colorectal Disease. 2005;7:304-310

[62] Leenen JPL, Hentzen JEKR, Ockhuijsen HDL. Effectiveness of mechanical bowel preparation versus no preparation on anastomotic leakage in colorectal surgery: A systematic review and meta- analysis. Updates in Surgery. 2019;**71**:227-236

[63] Guenaga KF, Matos D, Castro AA, Atallah AN, Wille-Jørgensen P. Mechanical bowel preparation for elective colorectal surgery. Cochrane Database of Systematic Reviews. Jan 25, 2005;(1):CD001544

[64] Jung B, Lannerstad O, Pahlman L, et al. Preoperative mechanical preparation of the colon: The patient's experience. BMC Surgery. 2007;**7**:5-9

[65] McSorley ST, Steele CW, McMahon AJ. Meta-analysis of oral antibiotics, in combination with preoperative intravenous antibiotics and mechanical bowel preparation the day before surgery, compared with intravenous antibiotics and mechanical bowel preparation alone to reduce surgical- site infections in elective colorectal surgery. BJS Open. 2018;**2**:185-194

[66] Rollins KE, Javanmard-Emamghissi H, Acheson AG, Lobo DN. The role of oral antibiotic preparation in elective colorectal surgery. Annals of Surgery. 2019;**270**(1):43-58

[67] Alcantara Moral M, Serra Aracil X, Bombardo Junca J, et al. A prospective, randomised, controlled study on the need to mechanically prepare the colon in scheduled colorectal surgery [in Spanish]. Cirugia Espanola. 2009;**85**:20-25

[68] Migaly J, Bafford AC, Francone TD, et al. American society of colon and rectal surgeons clinical practice guidelines for the use of bowel preparation in elective colon and rectal surgery. Diseases of the Colon & Rectum. 2019;**62**(1):3-8

[69] Zorbas KA, Yu D, Choudhry A, Ross HM, Philp M. Preoperative bowel preparation does not favor the management of colorectal anastomotic leak. World Journal of Gastrointestinal Surgery. 2019;**11**(4):218-228

[70] Nichols RL, Condon RE. Preoperative preparation of the colon. Surgery, Gynecology & Obstetrics. 1971;**132**:323-337

[71] Dellinger EP. Should a scheduled colorectal operation have a mechanical bowel prep, preoperative oral antibiotics, both, or neither? Annals of surgery. Lippincott Williams and Wilkins. 2015;**261**:1041-1043

[72] Smith MB, Goradia VK, Holmes JW, et al. Suppression of the human mucosal-related colonic microflora with

prophylactic parenteral and/or oral antibiotics. World Journal of Surgery. 1990;**14**:636-641

[73] Lewis RT. Oral versus systemic antibiotic prophylaxis in elective colon surgery: A randomized study and meta-analysis send a message from the 1990s. Canadian Journal of Surgery. 2002;**45**:173-180

[74] Markell KW, Hunt BM, Charron PD, et al. Prophylaxis and management of wound infection after elective colorectal surgery: A survey of the American Society of Colon and Rectal Surgeons membership. Journal of Gastrointestinal Surgery. 2010;**14**:1090e-11098e

[75] Golder AM, Steele CW, Conn D, et al. Effect of preoperative oral antibiotics in combination with mechanical bowel preparation on inflammatory response and short-term outcomes following left-sided colonic and rectal resections. BJS Open. 2019;**3**(6):830-839

[76] Kiran RP, ACA M, Chiuzan C, Estrada D, Forde K. Combined preoperative mechanical bowel preparation with oral antibiotics significantly reduces surgical site infection, anastomotic leak, and ileus after colorectal surgery. Annals of Surgery. 2015;**262**(3):416-425

[77] Wirth U, Rogers S, Haubensak K, et al. Local antibiotic decontamination to prevent anastomotic leakage short-term outcome in rectal cancer surgery. International Journal of Colorectal Disease. 2018;**33**:53-60

[78] Lee DS, Ryu JA, Chung CR, et al. Risk factors for acquisition of multidrug-resistant bacteria in patients with anastomotic leakage after colorectal cancer surgery. International Journal of Colorectal Disease. 2015;**30**:497-504

[79] Teillant A, Gandra S, Barter D, et al. Potential burden of antibiotic resistance on surgery and cancer chemotherapy antibiotic prophylaxis in the USA: A literature review and modelling study. Lancet Infectious Diseases. 2015;**15**:2429-2437

[80] Kirby A, Santoni N. Antibiotic resistance in Enterobacteriaceae: What impact on the efficacy of antibiotic prophylaxis in colorectal surgery? The Journal of Hospital Infection. 2015;**89**:259-263

[81] Clarke JS, Condon RE, Bartlett JG, et al. Preoperative oral antibiotics reduce septic complications of colon operations: Results of prospective, randomized, double-blind clinical study. Annals of Surgery. 1977;**186**:251-259

[82] Alverdy JC, Hyman N. Bowel preparation under siege. The British Journal of Surgery. 2020;**107**(3):167-170

[83] Rollins KE, Javanmard-Emamghissi H, Acheson AG, et al. The role of oral antibiotic preparation in elective colorectal surgery: A meta-analysis. Annals of Surgery. 2019;**270**:43-58

[84] Nichols RL, Gorbach SL, Condon RE. Alteration of intestinal microflora following preoperative mechanical preparation of the colon. Diseases of the Colon and Rectum. 1971;**14**(2):123-127

[85] Kim EK, Sheetz KH, Bonn J, et al. A state wide colectomy experience: The role of full bowel preparation in preventing surgical site infection. Annals of Surgery. 2014;**259**:310-314

[86] Garfinkle R, Abou Khalil J, Morin N, et al. Is there a role for oral antibiotic preparation alone before colorectal surgery? ACS-NSQIP analysis by coarsened exact matching. Diseases of the Colon and Rectum. 2017;**60**:729-737

[87] Leaper DJ, Edmiston CE. World Health Organization: Global guidelines for the prevention of surgical site infection. The Journal of Hospital Infection. 2017;**95**(2):135-136

[88] NICE. NICE—surgical site infections: prevention and treatment. 2019. https://www.nice.org.uk/guidance/cg74/resources/surgical-site-infections-prevention-and-treatment-975628422853

[89] Keenan JE, Speicher PJ, Thacker JK, Walter M, Kuchibhatla M, Mantyh CR. The preventive surgical site infection bundle in colorectal surgery: An effective approach to surgical site infection reduction and health care cost savings. JAMA Surgery. 2014;**149**:1045-1052

[90] Ohman KA, Wan L, Guthrie T, et al. Combination of oral antibiotics and mechanical bowel preparation reduces surgical site infection in colorectal surgery. Journal of the American College of Surgeons. 2017;**225**:465-471

[91] Ji WB, Hahn KY, Kwak JM, Kang DW, Baek SJ, Kim J, et al. Mechanical bowel preparation does not affect clinical severity of anastomotic leakage in rectal cancer surgery. World Journal of Surgery. 2017;**41**(5):1366-1374

[92] Bretagnol F, Panis Y, Rullier E, et al. Rectal cancer surgery with or without bowel preparation: The French GRECCAR III multi center single-blinded randomized trial. Annals of Surgery. 2010;**252**:863-868

[93] Mahajna A, Krausz M, Rosin D, et al. Bowel preparation is associated with spillage of bowel contents in colorectal surgery. Diseases of the Colon and Rectum. 2005;**48**:1626-1631

[94] Ikeda A, Konishi T, Ueno M, et al. Randomized clinical trial of oral and intravenous versus intravenous antibiotic prophylaxis for laparoscopic colorectal resection. The British Journal of Surgery. 2016;**103**:1608-1615

[95] Pittet O, Nocito A, Balke H, Duvoisin C, Clavien PA, Demartines N, et al. Rectal enema is an alternative to full mechanical bowel preparation for primary rectal cancer surgery. Colorectal Disease. 2015;**17**(11):1007-1010

[96] Gaynes RP, Culver DH, Horan TC, et al. Surgical site infection (SSI) rates in the United States, 1992-1998: The National Nosocomial Infections Surveillance System basic SSI risk index. Clinical Infectious Diseases. 2001;**33**(Suppl 2):S69-S77

[97] Siedhoff MT, Clark LH, Hobbs KA, Findley AD, Moulder JK, Garrett JM. Mechanical bowel preparation before laparoscopic hysterectomy: A randomized controlled trial. Obstetrics and Gynecology. 2014;**123**(3):562-567

[98] Yang LC, Arden D, Lee TT, Mansuria SM, Broach AN, D'Ambrosio L, et al. Mechanical bowel preparation for gynecologic laparoscopy: A prospective randomized trial of oral sodium phosphate solution vs single sodium phosphate enema. Journal of Minimally Invasive Gynecology. 2011;**18**(2):149-156

[99] Mulayim B, Karadag B. Do we need mechanical bowel preparation before benign gynecologic laparoscopic surgeries a randomized, single-blind, controlled trial. Gynecologic and Obstetric Investigation. 2018;**83**(2):203-208

[100] Zmora O, Lebedyev A, Hoffman A, Khaikin M, Munz Y, Shabtai M, et al. Laparoscopic colectomy without mechanical bowel preparation. International Journal of Colorectal Disease. 2006;**21**(7):683-687

[101] Chan MY, Foo CC, Poon JTC, Law WL. Laparoscopic colorectal resections with and without routine mechanical bowel preparation: A comparative study. Annals of Medicine and Surgery. 2016 Aug;**1**(9):72-76

[102] Vlot J, Slieker JC, Wijnen R, Lange JF, Bax KN. Optimizing working-space in laparoscopy: Measuring the effect of mechanical bowel preparation in a porcine model. Surgical Endoscopy. 2013;**27**(6):1980-1985

[103] Won H, Maley P, Salim S, Rao A, Campbell NT, Abbott JA. Surgical and patient outcomes using mechanical bowel preparation before laparoscopic gynecologic surgery: A randomized controlled trial. Obstetrics and Gynecology. 2013;**121**(3):538-546

[104] Drummond RJ, McKenna RM, Wright DM. Current practice in bowel preparation for colorectal surgery: A survey of the members of the Association of Coloproctology of GB & Ireland. Colorectal Disease. 2011;**13**(6):708-710

[105] Andersen J, Thorup J, Wille-Jørgensen P. Use of preoperative bowel preparation in elective colorectal surgery in Denmark remains high. Danish Medical Bulletin. 2011;**58**(9):A4313

[106] Lohsiriwat V, Lohsiriwat D, Thavichaigarn P. Current practices in rectal cancer surgery: A survey of Thai colorectal surgeons. Journal of the Medical Association of Thailand. 2009;**92**(8):1009-1015

[107] Vignali A, Gianotti L, Braga M, et al. Altered microperfusion at the rectal stump is predictive for rectal anastomotic leak. Diseases of the Colon and Rectum. 2000;**43**:76-82

[108] Shakhsheer BA, Lec B, Zaborin A, et al. Lack of evidence for tissue hypoxia as a contributing factor in anastomotic leak following colon anastomosis and segmental devascularization in rats. International Journal of Colorectal Disease. 2016;**32**(4):539-547

[109] Ringel Y, Maharshak N, Ringel-Kulka T, et al. High throughput sequencing reveals distinct microbial populations within the mucosal and luminal niches in healthy individuals. Gut Microbes. 2015;**6**(3):173-181

[110] van der Beek CM, Dejong CHC, Troost FJ, et al. Role of short-chain fatty acids in colonic inflammation, carcinogenesis, and mucosal protection and healing. Nutrition Reviews. 2017;**75**(4):286-305

[111] Alam A, Leoni G, Quiros M, et al. The microenvironment of injured murine gut elicits a local pro-restitutive microbiota. Nature Microbiology. 2016;**1**:15021

[112] Alverdy JC, Hyman N, Gilbert J, Luo JN, Krezalek M. Preparing the bowel for surgery: Learning from the past and planning for the future. Journal of the American College of Surgeons. 2017;**225**(2):324-332

[113] Gaines S, Shao C, Hyman N, Alverdy JC. Gut microbiome influences on anastomotic leak and recurrence rates following colorectal cancer surgery. The British Journal of Surgery. 2018;**105**(2):e131-e141

[114] Konishi T, Watanabe T, Kishimoto J, et al. Elective colon and rectal surgery differ in risk factors for wound infection: Results of prospective surveillance. Annals of Surgery. 2006;**244**:758-763

[115] Toh JWT, Phan K, Hitos K, Pathma-Nathan N, El-Khoury T, Richardson AJ, et al. Association of Mechanical Bowel Preparation and Oral

Antibiotics before Elective Colorectal Surgery with surgical site infection: A network meta-analysis. JAMA Network Open. 2018;**1**(6):e183226

[116] Ambe PC, Zarras K, Stodolski M, Wirjawan I, Zirngibl H. Routine preoperative mechanical bowel preparation with additive oral antibiotics is associated with a reduced risk of anastomotic leakage in patients undergoing elective oncologic resection for colorectal cancer. World Journal of Surgical Oncology. 2019;**17**(1):20

[117] Murphy MM, Tevis SE, Kennedy GD. Independent risk factors for prolonged postoperative ileus development. The Journal of Surgical Research. 2016;**201**(2):279-285

[118] Althumairi AA, Canner JK, Pawlik TM, Schneider E, Nagarajan N, Safar B, et al. Benefits of bowel preparation beyond surgical site infection: A retrospective study. Annals of Surgery. 2016;**264**(6):1051-1057

Chapter 8

Post-Prostatectomy Urinary Incontinence

Filippo Marino, Francesco Rossi and Emilio Sacco

Abstract

Post-prostatectomy urinary incontinence (PPUI) represents the most bothersome long-term complication of prostatectomy. While the risk of PPUI due to invasive treatments of benign prostatic hyperplasia appears to be low (about 1%), the risk is significantly higher after radical prostatectomy (10–50%). Although both external urethral sphincter deficiency and bladder dysfunctions have been considered responsible for PPUI, sphincter deficiency is the most important determinant. Fortunately, PPUI can be effectively cured by specialized management. The first-line treatment based on pelvic floor muscle training has been shown to accelerate continence recovery. Duloxetine is the only available medical treatment demonstrating clinical efficacy for mild-to-moderate PPUI. However, side effects commonly lead to 15–31% of withdrawal. As a result, in the case of refractory PPUI, more invasive options are recommended including artificial urinary sphincters and male slings. Level 1 evidence has been achieved on the efficacy of these surgical treatments that need to be indicated based on an accurate preoperative workout and shared decision-making.

Keywords: incontinence, male urinary incontinence, radical prostatectomy, post-prostatectomy urinary incontinence, prostate cancer

1. Introduction

Prostate cancer is the most common tumor among men. It has a strong genetic component and is the second most diagnosed tumor worldwide after lung cancer [1, 2]. Radical prostatectomy (RP) and radiation beam therapy represent comparable treatment options for localized disease [3].

One of the major complications of RP is urinary incontinence (UI), with a notoriously negative impact on the patient's quality of life (QoL) and daily activities [4]. UI is the complaint of any involuntary loss of urine [5], with a prevalence of 11–34% in older men [6, 7]. The occurrence of post-prostatectomy urinary incontinence (PPUI) rate varies from 5 to 40% [8] up to 69% [9], depending on the series of patients examined. These differences in PPUI incidence have been attributed to the surgeon's experience, surgical technique, length of follow-up, data acquisition methods, and differing continence definitions [10]. Current definitions of continence vary from no leakage at all, no pads use but loss of few drops of urine [11], or the use of no more than 1 pad per day, defined as social continence [12].

The etiology of PPUI is often multifactorial and may depend on the patient's characteristics, sphincteric competence, anatomic support, pelvic innervation, and technical surgical factors such as extensive dissection, neurovascular bundle damage, and the development of postoperative fibrosis [13]. Several risk factors have been reported, including greater age at surgery, obesity, shorter membranous urethral length (MUL), prostate volume, prior transurethral resection of the prostate (TURP), bladder dysfunction, tumor stage and no nerve-sparing surgery [8, 14].

The most common type of PPUI is stress urinary incontinence (SUI), which consists of involuntary leakage during exertion, sneezing, or coughing [5].

Overactive bladder syndrome (OAB) with urge urinary incontinence can also occur after RP. The underlying mechanisms are still under debate, with an outlined hypothesis of detrusor overactivity due to partial bladder denervation during prostate surgery [13].

Continence status continues to evolve from more than 1 year after RP and about 80% of incontinent patients regain continence status without direct treatment [15]. Conservative strategies for the management of PPUI should be trialed as a first option before proceeding to more invasive options. The most common conservative treatments include behavioral therapy, pelvic floor muscle training (PFMT) with or without biofeedback, electronic stimulation, and pharmacotherapy [16]. When these options fail, surgical management is the treatment of choice with artificial urinary sphincter and male sling implantation.

2. Pathophysiology and anatomic components

The pathophysiology of PPUI has yet to be entirely understood. However, numerous theories have been proposed. Pelvic support and neuromuscular anatomic components have been recognized as significant contributing factors to PPUI [17]. Biological and preoperative factors such as age, high BMI, preexisting lower urinary tract symptoms (LUTS), prostate size, short MUL, and functional bladder alterations have a negative impact on continence status after RP [14].

2.1 Direct damage to the urethral sphincter complex

The urethral sphincter's complex, which extends from the vesical orifice to the perineal membrane, comprises an internal sphincter (lissosphincter) made of smooth muscle and an external sphincter (rhabdosphincter) made of skeletal muscle [18]. During everyday activities, when there is minimal strain on the bladder outflow, the internal sphincter is responsible for maintaining continence (passive continence). It sustains tone for an extended time with little effort [14, 18]. On the other hand, the external sphincter is responsible for continence under stress (active continence). It comprises slow and fast twitch fibers that allow a tonic contraction for baseline continence and temporary recruitment in response to rapid pressure rise and/or voluntary blockage of the urine flow [18, 19].

Preservation of the internal sphincter is believed to be achievable through bladder neck-sparing surgery. The preservation of the internal sphincter complex has been observed to lead to a quicker return to continence and a reduced incidence of postoperative incontinence [20, 21]. However, Marien and Lepor [22] showed that sparing the bladder neck does not significantly impact continence rates. Furthermore, bladder neck preservation may increase the risk of positive surgical margins in case of a tumor located at the prostatic base.

External urethral sphincter deficiency is considered the most important determinant of PPUI [23]. Transurethral ultrasound examination has revealed thinning or atrophy, and compromised contractility [24]. Sphincteric incontinence is the urodynamic measurement's most common finding [25].

The contribution of neurovascular bundles (NVBs) in the innervation of the external urethral rhabdosphincter is a topic of ongoing debate. At the same time, the effect of NVB preservation during RP on erectile function is evident [26]. Some authors believe that NVB damage affects the continence mechanism and that preservation leads to at least an earlier continence recovery after surgery [20, 27–29]. However, other authors found no difference in continence rates between nerve-sparing and nonnerve-sparing techniques [22]. Recent results from a randomized clinical trial (IMPROVE trial, NCT02367404) [30] of 240 men with organ-confined prostate cancer who underwent RP, demonstrated that NVB preservation was the only factor associated with continence recovery.

2.2 Damage to the supporting structures of the membranous urethra

The male urethra's supporting structures can be divided into the anterior and posterior supporting structures and the pelvic floor (levator ani muscle). The pubovesical, puboprostatic ligaments and the tendinous arch of the pelvic fascia form the anterior urethral support structures. The ligaments stabilize the location of the bladder neck and the membranous urethra to the pubic bone [31]. The posterior support comprises the central perineal tendon, the Denonvilliers' fascia, and the rectourethralis muscle [32]. The third support structure includes the levator ani muscle and surrounding fascia [33]. The pelvic floor is not directly connected to the urethra, but it contributes to continence by exerting an occlusive force on the urethra via increased intra-abdominal pressure [33, 34].

PPUI can be improved by maintaining the integrity of the puboprostatic and pubovesical ligaments, allowing proper sphincter functioning [35, 36]. Several studies have demonstrated that the reconstruction of the posterior musculofascial plate of Denonvilliers (also known as the *Rocco stitch*) appears to improve PPUI [36–38]. However, some surgeons did not observe a similar improvement in continence after RP [22]. Total pelvic reconstruction with anterior and posterior fixation and anchoring of the bladder urethra anastomosis and the sphincteric complex appear to improve biomechanics and continence [36]. Like the Rocco stitch, this technique prevents urethral stump recession [37] and reduces anastomosis tension, improving mucosal coaptation. However, definitive evidence of their efficacy in the prevention of long-term PPUI still needs to be identified.

Due to the anatomical complexities of the structures surrounding the prostate gland, the surgeon's experience level is one of the most significant determinants of successful outcomes. The primary intraoperative and postoperative mechanisms of injuries are summarized in **Table 1** [24].

2.3 Detrusor dysfunctions

Detrusor dysfunctions have been attributed to postoperative bladder decentralization, inflammation and/or infection, and geometric bladder wall alteration linked to preexisting hypoxemia with/without neuroplasticity [39]. Detrusor dysfunction was infrequently a single diagnosis and was typically accompanied by intrinsic sphincteric dysfunction. Surgical damage to the pudendal nerve fibers that innervate the

Intraoperative injuries			Postoperative injuries
Muscle injuries	**Nerves injuries**	**Supporting structures injuries**	
Direct damage during apical dissection	Neurovascular bundles resection	Cutting of puboprostatic ligaments	Urethral fibrosis due to devascularization and/or radiotherapy
Electrocautery	Hypogastric plexus damage during lymphadenectomy	Cutting of posterior urethral attachments (Denonvillier's fascia)	Disordered reinnervation
Hemostatic and anastomotic sutures	Electrocautery and tractions, bladder mobilization	Disruption of endopelvic fascia	Bladder neck strictures and incision
Devascularization	Anastomotic sutures at 5–7 o'clock	Detachment from perineal body	Hemostatic clips erosion and extrusion

Table 1.
Intraoperative and postoperative injuries directly or indirectly affecting external urethral sphincter function.

rhabdosphincter has functional consequences. In 2–77% of patients, detrusor overactivity was a *de novo* dysfunction. Patients with impaired bladder compliance ranged from 8 to 39%, with approximately 50% of cases being *de novo*. Detrusor hypocontractility was observed in 29–61% of patients, was *de novo* in 47%, and recovered in about 50% of patients [39].

Detrusor contractility may be impaired during surgery. Postoperative detrusor underactivity following RP seems to be an irreversible phenomenon persisting even over the long term [40].

3. Diagnostic evaluation

A comprehensive assessment typically begins with a detailed medical history, physical examination, and an objective assessment of symptoms.

The medical history should focus on the type, timing, and severity of incontinence throughout the day, the presence or absence of nighttime and gravitational incontinence, and the presence of incontinence-triggering situations (e.g., straining, coughing, or sneezing). The history should also assess any preexisting LUTS, details regarding the prostatectomy procedure, comorbidities, prior radiotherapy, interventions for urethral strictures or incontinence, and the oncological status [41].

The physical evaluation should include an abdominal, neuro-urological, and perineal examination, as well as a digital rectal examination. Furthermore, manual dexterity should be assessed before an artificial urinary sphincter (AUS) implantation, which requires manipulation of the activating pump [42].

Micturition time charts and bladder diaries are standardized tools for measuring and monitoring symptom severity, evaluating the frequency, number of incontinence episodes, voided volumes, and 24-h urinary output [43]. Available validated questionnaires include the International Consultation on Incontinence-Short Form [44] and the UCLA/RAND-Prostate Cancer Index Urinary Function Score [45], which are the most frequently used. Patients' subjective perception of how much they leak is unreliable; therefore, objective measures should be required for evaluation [46]. Pad count appears to be a poor measure of the degree of UI due to limitations such as different sizes, pad absorbency, and degree of saturation [47, 48]. On the other hand, pad weight is recognized as the most accurate metric for UI assessment [47]. Evidence indicates that the 24-h and 48-h pad weighing tests are the most accurate for quantifying and diagnosing UI severity [47, 49].

The primary diagnostic should be performed before scheduling initial conservative treatment, including urinalysis to rule out infection and bladder ultrasound to assess postvoid residual urine volume [41].

If this attempt fails and surgical treatment is planned, a more invasive diagnosis should be performed [41]. Urethrocystoscopy aims to rule out urethral pathologies, such as bladder neck stenosis or urethral stricture, that may complicate a future surgical approach. Urethroscopy can also be used to perform the *repositioning test,* which consists of applying gentle mid-perineal pressure parallel to the anal canal while a 0° cystoscope is positioned distally of the sphincter region, and a view of the entire circumference of the external urinary sphincter is obtained. The test yields a positive result when the sphincter autonomously and reflexively closes concentrically, exhibiting complete closure during the repositioning of the posterior urethra [50]. This evaluation is essential in determining the patient's residual sphincter function and determines suitability for potential retrourethral sling implantation [50].

A urodynamic test is required if the patient has neurogenic disorders or OAB symptoms, especially to assess detrusor function [51]. However, the use of urodynamics in therapeutic decision-making is still debated. As reported by some authors, a higher preoperative Valsalva Leak Point Pressure (VLPP) (>70 cm H_2O or > 100 cm H_2O) better predicts successful outcomes for male sling implantation [52, 53]. In contrast, Han et al. found no negative impact of an impaired preoperative VLPP on functional outcomes after male sling placement [54]. In patients undergoing artificial urinary sphincter implantation due to intrinsic sphincter deficiency, there was no correlation between preoperative urodynamic findings and surgical outcomes [55]. Recent evidence indicates that the urodynamic study might not be relevant in all PPUI patients [56].

Urethrocystography may be a valuable supplementary diagnostic tool in cases suspicious of urethra abnormalities to rule out or better characterize a urethral stricture or bladder neck contracture [57].

4. Treatment options

4.1 Conservative and pharmacological treatments

After RP, improvements in continence status will evolve from the early postoperative period until the end of the first year [8, 58]. Before proceeding to more invasive treatments, conservative management should be evaluated, and patients should be monitored regularly to determine the degree of improvement [16]. The most common conservative treatments are lifestyle interventions, physiotherapy (PFMT) with or without biofeedback or electrical stimulation, and pharmacotherapy.

Lifestyle interventions include time voiding or double voiding, fluid restriction, smoking cessation, and reducing bladder irritants (caffeine, alcohol, hot spices) [16, 41].

PFMT consists of a program of repeated voluntary pelvic floor muscle contractions to improve the closure mechanism due to the levator ani muscle [59, 60]. According to the current European Association of Urology (EAU) guidelines, PFMT should be offered to all patients undergoing RP to speed up postoperative continence recovery [41]. Debate on combining PFMT with additional biofeedback training or electrical stimulation is ongoing. Current evidence supporting PFMT with or without biofeedback is conflicting; some randomized trials demonstrated improved continence thanks to biofeedback therapy [61], and others indicated no benefit [62]. Based on 7th International Consultation on Incontinence (ICI), to achieve a significant improvement, PFMT should be performed for at least 3 months from RP and should be offered for periods of up to 6–12 months [63]. Evidence suggests that electrical stimulation may accelerate urinary continence recovery, but no long-term benefit has been demonstrated at 6 months or more after surgery [64].

Regarding pharmacologic treatments, no approved drugs yet exist. Antimuscarinics, phosphodiesterase inhibitors, and alpha-adrenergic agonists have been proposed as potential therapies for PPUI, especially in patients with OAB symptoms, demonstrating unexciting results [65].

Duloxetine, a serotonin-noradrenaline reuptake inhibitor, is the only available medical treatment that showed clinical efficacy for mild-to-moderate PPUI, increasing the neural tone of the urethral sphincter to prevent incontinent episodes [66, 67]. It has been approved for female stress urinary incontinence in some countries, but there is evidence that it reduces SUI-related symptoms in males [68, 69]. Gastrointestinal and central nervous side effects are common, leading to 15–31% of withdrawal [70]. These side effects are usually limited to the initial phase, and the use of duloxetine can be efficacious with persistence [71]. Some authors showed that duloxetine has synergistic effects when combined with PFMT [72]. However, clinical evidence supporting their routine use is weak. These two treatments seem to improve early continence recovery moderately, but neither significantly improves long-term urinary continence [73]. Recent results from a randomized clinical trial by Sanchez-Salas et al. demonstrated that PFMT and duloxetine do not improve urinary continence recovery, may have a negative impact on quality of life, and should not be routinely recommended to patients after RP [30].

In the case of refractory PPUI, more invasive and effective options are recommended.

4.2 Surgical treatments

If conservative therapy fails, surgical treatment options should be offered. Invasive treatment options include peri-urethral balloons, bulking agents, artificial urinary sphincters (AUS), and male slings.

AUS and perineal slings are the most used surgical treatment options. European guidelines recommend the AUS implantation for patients with moderate-to-severe PPUI after unsuccessful conservative treatment. Conversely, for mild-to-moderate PPUI, fixed perineal slings are recommended [74]. As a result, moderate urinary incontinence is in a "grey area" in which both AUS and slings are indicated, despite growing evidence that AUS significantly outperforms fixed slings in men with moderate PPUI [75].

Peri-urethral balloons can be considered a salvage therapy for mild, persistent, or recurrent PPUI after implantation of a fixed male sling [74].

4.2.1 Artificial urinary sphincter

The AUS was conceptualized and created by F. Brantley Scott in 1973 [76]. The original AMS 721 model has undergone several modifications and enhancements, leading to the current model AMS 800® (Boston Scientific, Boston, MA, USA), which is the currently established standard for managing moderate to severe PPUI [77]. The AUS comprises a urethral cuff, a pressure-regulating balloon (PRB), and a pump. It is a hydraulic, mechanical device functioning through a circumferential compression of the urethra. The PRB and the cuff come, with different pressure ranges and sizes, respectively, to adapt the device to the patient's characteristics.

After five decades since its introduction, a considerable number of cohort studies have demonstrated the efficacy and reliability of AUS in terms of continence and quality-of-life improvement [77]. However, significant limitations to AUS use include the device's mechanical nature, which necessitates adequate manual dexterity and cognition, the persistent need for some pad use in many patients, the worries over potential complications, the need for reoperation due to mechanical failure in about a third of patients, and costs. Consequently, patients should be really motivated for the implantation and informed about the risk of future reoperations.

At our institution, patient preparation is performed following an internal protocol. Antiseptic washing is performed the day before surgery, and trichotomy is done just before surgery. Patients are placed in a high lithotomy position, and chlorhexidine gluconate abdominal and perineal scrub (10 min) is performed. An abdominal-perineal dual-surgical approach is usually used. We implemented a standardized protocol for asepsis to avoid infection, including minimization of operating room traffic, dual single-shot antibiotic prophylaxis (cephazolin and gentamicin), minimum air exposure of the device component, use of double gloves by the members of the surgical team with frequent gloves changes, as well as rinsing of the operative field and PRB with antibiotic solution, use of medicated drapes to isolate skin, meticulous hemostasis, and minimization of tissue dissection. A 12 Fr transurethral catheter is used. In cases of bladder neck contracture, patients are preferentially treated by adopting a two-stage approach with an endoscopic incision performed before the AUS implantation. We usually transpose the cuff tube at the abdominal level and suture the perineum at this point of the procedure to minimize air exposure. The PRB (61–70 cmH2O) is placed intraperitoneally through a McBurney incision, and the pump is implanted in the scrotum. At the end of the procedure, the system is cycled twice, and the pump is deactivated. Skin incisions are approximated with adsorbable running intradermal sutures. The bladder catheter is removed on postoperative day two. Patients are discharged on day three, and the urinary sphincter is activated 6 weeks later [78].

PRB placement has evolved. Some surgeons place it in the space of Retzius. This location has rarely been associated with serious complications, given its proximity to the bowel and bladder. Other authors suggested an alternative ectopic PRB placement via a counter incision in the anterior abdominal wall [79]. Balloon herniation, palpability, and pain represent a possible bothersome complication of the aforementioned locations, thereby, we utilize a deeper pelvic location (intraperitoneally) through a suprainguinal incision.

In clinical practice, one may encounter situations (previous radiotherapy, previous UI surgery, etc.) requiring a different surgical approach.

The bulbar urethra at the level of the bifurcation of the corporal bodies is the most frequently used site for AUS cuff implantation [80]. A distal single or double cuff placement is commonly required in patients undergoing AUS reimplantation following urethral erosion or in those with urethral atrophy at the original cuff site [81]. In cases of compromised urethra due to prior AUS placement, previous radiation therapy, or urethral surgery, the AUS cuff may be placed through a transcorporal approach that protects the posterior wall of the urethra during dissection to decrease the risk of urethral lesions or erosion [82]. The risk of impaired erectile function due to disruption of the tunica albuginea of the corporal bodies is the major drawback of the transcorporal approach that limits its widespread use [83].

The AMS 800 remains the gold standard treatment for PPUI, offering a very satisfactory and predictable continence rate and high patient satisfaction.

Definitions of continence based on pad use are heterogenous in the literature; however, in AUS publications, the "social continence, defined as the use of, at maximum, one pad per day, is the most used quantitative functional outcome." Van der Aa et al. reported a social continence rate of 79.0% (60.9–100%) [77].

However, AUS implantation is associated with a likely underreported risk of intraoperative urethral lesions and postoperative urethral erosions [77]. The data about infection and erosion rates after AUS placement are inconsistent, with most papers not reporting the erosion and the infection rates separately, counting them as a composite outcome. In a pooled analysis [77] of 12 studies, the mean infection plus erosion rate was 8.5% (3.3–27.8%).

Based on the bi-layered structure with multiple sublayers of the tunica albuginea of the corpora cavernosa, we assessed an alternative "*transalbugineal*" AUS implantation technique intending to decrease perioperative morbidity while preserving the integrity of the corpora cavernosa [78]. After identifying and splitting the bulbospongiosus muscle, the corpus spongiosum is gently exposed in its anterolateral aspect. Buck's fascia is incised bilaterally, and the posterior dissection is performed starting 5 mm off the bulbar urethra on both sides, entering the multilayered structure of the tunica albuginea of the corpora cavernosa, thus leaving its external layer attached to the posterior aspect of the urethra. The main aim of our modified technique was to reduce the risk of intraoperative urethral injuries and the risk of postoperative urethral erosion (and consequent infection) due to shallow dissection, without compromising sexual function in potent patients. Our refined implantation technique was demonstrated to be effective, safe, and reproducible, with continence rates similar to those achieved using a conventional approach.

Further potential complications consist of both mechanical and nonmechanical failures, which can manifest as either early or late postoperative complications and may necessitate reoperation. The most common causes of surgical revision are pump migration or malfunction, liquid leakage from the connector, infection, urethral erosion, and urethral atrophy.

Overall, the AUS survival rate is around 90% at 1 year, 57% at 10 years, and 41% at 15 years [84]. A pooled analysis of complications showed mechanical failure in 6.2%, urethral atrophy in 7.9%, and a global reoperation rate for any reason in 26.0% of patients [77]. Urethral erosion or device infection typically results in AUS explantation. A second device implant is associated with a worse outcome [85].

Several competing devices have been introduced in recent years, including the VICTO (Promodon, Cordoba, Argentina) and the Zephyr ZSI 375 (Mayor Group, Villeurbanne, France) systems.

VICTO is an adjustable preconnected AUS. A small silicone balloon regulates the pressure in the occluding cuff, and the control pump has a self-sealing port for pressure adjustment [86]. The system pressure can be adjusted from 0 to 100 cm of water. VICTO +, with an additional stress balloon placed in the preperitoneal region, is available for patients who were unable to interrupt the stream. Thereby, abdominal pressure changes are directly transferred to the urethral cuff [87].

Zephyr ZSI 375 is another all-in-one silicone-elastomeric device [88], without an abdominal reservoir and with an inflatable cuff in which pressure can be adjusted by instilling or abolishing fluid. Neither device is currently approved for use in the US.

4.2.2 Male slings

Male slings are polypropylene meshes positioned over the bulbar urethra via transobturator route [89]. The concept of the male sling was initially proposed by Berry in the 1970s and subsequently refined by Kaufman and Schaefer, resulting in the current medical device used in clinical practice [90]. Slings cure urinary incontinence by simple urethral compression and/or bulb repositioning to restore the preprostatectomy configuration of the prolapsed urethral sphincter complex [91].

Synthetic male slings are becoming increasingly common because they are reasonably inexpensive and do not require mechanical manipulation when voiding. Most experienced urologists recognize that selecting the correct patient is essential for successful treatment. Patients with mild-to-moderate SUI and adequate residual sphincter function, which allows for enough detrusor contraction to overcome the fixed sling impediment and allow voiding, are the best candidates [92].

Male slings are classified as adjustable and nonadjustable based on whether the tension can be adjusted or not after the procedure according to the patient's continence status [51].

Commercially available adjustable male slings are Argon (Promedon, Cordoba, Argentina), Re-Meex (Neomedic, Barcelona, Spain), and ATOMS (AMI, Feldkirch, Austria), while current nonadjustable male slings are AdVance (Boston Scientific, Minnetonka, MN, USA), I-STOP TOMS (CL Medical, Lyon, France), and Virtue (Coloplast, Minneapolis, MN, USA).

There are no studies that compare individual devices. As a result, determining the success rate of operations is difficult, and judging which sling system is superior is challenging [93].

AdVance XP sling is the evolution of AdVance sling (Boston Scientific, Marlborough, MA, USA), a retrourethral sling that contains polypropylene mesh. It is placed via a transobturator approach around the proximal bulbar urethra. To accurately position the sling, the central tendon of the perineum must be released. The mesh is then attached to the bulbous urethra, and the tension is applied so that the membranous urethra can be relocated further proximally. Continence is achieved through a 3–4 cm proximal elevation of the bulbar urethra [94].

The AdVance XP model, launched in 2010, has improved stability due to tensioning fibers, chevron anchors, and Tyvek (DuPont, Wilmington, DE, USA) liners. Furthermore, the implantation needle was modified to facilitate placement [95].

In our practice, we utilize a bulbospongiosus muscle-sparing surgical technique for the insertion of the AdVanceXP sling, with the aim to decrease postoperative complications (acute urinary retention and urethral erosion) [96]. The muscle-sparing approach consists of placing the sling directly on the bulbospongiosus muscle, unlike the standard technique, which requires the opening of the bulbospongiosus muscle and the placing of the sling on the underlying corpus spongiosum. The preservation of an intact and healthy proximal bulbar urethra is particularly desirable in failed patients requiring subsequent AUS implantation [96].

There is level 1 evidence that male sling can cure or improve PPUI with an overall success rate between 60 and 80% [97, 98]. Success is inversely correlated with SUI severity, with mild incontinence achieving success rates of 80–90%, even outperforming the AUS [99]. However, for those with moderate SUI, the AUS outperforms the sling, with sling success rates ranging from 32 to 83% [48, 75]. The severity of SUI has been associated with worse outcomes; therefore, patient selection is the key to success [94].

Failure rates after sling placement range from 15 to 45% and current knowledge of predictors of sling efficacy is limited [100].

Literature reports a postoperative complication rate ranging from 1 to 45% [101]. Perineal pain is the most common complaint, with an estimated rate as high as 45%. Urinary retention rates range from 2 to 23%, depending on the type of sling selected. Other uncommon complications include urethral erosion and infection. Revision rates are reported at approximately 1% [93, 94].

A recent noninferiority randomized controlled trial compared synthetic slings with AUS. The former was comparable to the latter in terms of continence rate improvements, symptoms, quality of life, and treatment-related satisfaction [98].

4.2.3 Peri-urethral balloons

The ProACT® (Uromedica, Inc., Plymouth, MN, USA) is a noncircumferential compressive device consisting of two silicone balloons that are implanted by a trocar via two small perineal incisions and are placed under fluoroscopic guidance on each side of the bladder neck, close to the vesicourethral anastomotic site. An outpatient procedure fills the balloons, resulting in mechanical compression of the urethra [102].

The potential benefits of the ProACT device include technical reliability of implantation, low morbidity, a low price, the absence of circumferential urethral compression, and the possibility to modulate the degree of urethral compression [103].

The efficacy is reported to be 55% (30–75%), but more than a third of patients were not satisfied with the outcome of the surgery [104]. The success rates are negatively impacted by the severity of incontinence and a prior history of radiation therapy, which some authors consider a contraindication [74, 105].

There is currently no direct recommendation in the European guidelines for using ProACT. These device implantations should be exclusively performed at specialized centers due to the specific surgical technique, the complexity of indications, and the potential risks of erosion, mechanical failure, and subsequent reoperation, with an estimated explantation rate of 25% [74].

4.2.4 Bulking agents

In patients with PPUI persistent and refractory to conservative management or in patients unfit for more invasive surgical treatment, bulking agents are an option that can be chosen [106].

Among all the bulking agents, polytetrafluoroethylene (Teflon) and bovine collagen have been the first two agents used. More recent elements are represented by adipose tissue (1989) and stem cells (2007) [107].

Based on a systematic review by Toia et al. [106], bulking agents can improve continence rates, at least in the short term.

Bulking agents are injected endoscopically into the sphincteric complex, increasing the sphincter's coaptation and resistance to flow [65]. A controversy exists on injection volume and site, leading to variable functional improvements between different centers [106].

According to a recent meta-analysis, which compared the different devices used for treating PPUI, bulking agents are associated with the lowest improvement in continence after treatment. In addition, the more the injections are, the lower the continence rates and improvements are [108].

5. Conclusion

PPUI is not an infrequent event that negatively impacts a patient's quality of life and is related to considerable economic pressure. A wide range of treatment options is available, ranging from conservative methods to invasive surgical procedures.

PFMT is suggested for the initial management of PPUI, while anticholinergic drugs are used for urgent symptoms.

AUS was the preferred treatment for patients with consistent PPUI for several decades. Male slings are currently becoming a valuable alternative for patients with mild-to-moderate PPUI. A meticulous preoperative workup should be conducted when planning a male PPUI surgery and the surgical approach should be chosen based on the disease's severity. Patients with an unclear or inconsistent history should undergo further objective workup, including cystoscopy and/or urodynamics. Ongoing research will help to stratify patients and sustain preoperative decision-making.

Author details

Filippo Marino*, Francesco Rossi and Emilio Sacco
Urology Department, Agostino Gemelli Academic Hospital Foundation IRCCS, Catholic University School of Medicine of Rome, Rome, Italy

*Address all correspondence to: dr.filippomarino@gmail.com

References

[1] Siegel RL, Miller KD, Fuchs HE, et al. Cancer statistics, 2022. CA: A Cancer Journal for Clinicians. 2022;**72**(1):7-33. DOI: 10.3322/caac.21708

[2] Marino F, Totaro A, Gandi C, et al. Germline mutations in prostate cancer: A systematic review of the evidence for personalized medicine. Prostate Cancer and Prostatic Diseases. 2022. DOI: 10.1038/s41391-022-00609-3 [Online ahead of print]

[3] Mottet N, Cornford P, Van Den Bergh RCN, et al. European Association of Urology (EAU) Guidelines on Management of Prostate Cancer. 2023. Available from: https://uroweb.org/guidelines/prostate-cancer [Accessed: June 2023]

[4] Sanda MG, Dunn RL, Michalski J, et al. Quality of life and satisfaction with outcome among prostate-cancer survivors. The New England Journal of Medicine. 2008;**358**(12):1250-1261. DOI: 10.1056/NEJMoa074311

[5] D'Ancona C, Haylen B, Oelke M, et al. The international continence society (ICS) report on the terminology for adult male lower urinary tract and pelvic floor symptoms and dysfunction. Neurourology and Urodynamics. 2019;**38**(2):433-477. DOI: 10.1002/nau.23897

[6] Boyle P, Robertson C, Mazzetta C, et al. The prevalence of male urinary incontinence in four centres: The UREPIK study. BJU International. 2003;**92**(9):943-947. DOI: 10.1111/j.1464-410x.2003.04526.x

[7] Shamliyan TA, Wyman JF, Ping R, et al. Male urinary incontinence: Prevalence, risk factors, and preventive interventions. Revista de Urología. 2009;**11**(3):145-165

[8] Sacco E, Prayer-Galetti T, Pinto F, et al. Urinary incontinence after radical prostatectomy: Incidence by definition, risk factors and temporal trend in a large series with a long-term follow-up. BJU International. 2006;**97**(6):1234-1241. DOI: 10.1111/j.1464-410X.2006.06185.x

[9] Wei JT, Dunn RL, Marcovich R, et al. Prospective assessment of patient reported urinary continence after radical prostatectomy. The Journal of Urology. 2000;**164**(3 Pt 1):744-748. DOI: 10.1097/00005392-200009010-00029

[10] Trost L, Elliott DS. Male stress urinary incontinence: A review of surgical treatment options and outcomes. Advances in Urology. 2012;**2012**:287489. DOI: 10.1155/2012/287489

[11] Nitti VW, Mourtzinos A, Brucker BM, et al. Correlation of patient perception of pad use with objective degree of incontinence measured by pad test in men with post-prostatectomy incontinence: The SUFU pad test study. The Journal of Urology. 2014;**192**(3):836-842. DOI: 10.1016/j.juro.2014.03.031

[12] James MH, McCammon KA. Artificial urinary sphincter for post-prostatectomy incontinence: A review. International Journal of Urology. 2014;**21**(6):536-543. DOI: 10.1111/iju.12392

[13] Rahnama'i MS, Marcelissen T, Geavlete B, et al. Current Management of Post-radical Prostatectomy Urinary Incontinence. Frontiers in Surgery. 2021;**8**:647656. DOI: 10.3389/fsurg.2021.647656

[14] Heesakkers J, Farag F, Bauer RM, et al. Pathophysiology and contributing

factors in Postprostatectomy incontinence: A review. European Urology. 2017;**71**(6):936-944. DOI: 10.1016/j.eururo.2016.09.031

[15] Litwin MS, Melmed GY, Nakazon T. Life after radical prostatectomy: A longitudinal study. The Journal of Urology. 2001;**166**(2):587-592

[16] Sountoulides P, Vakalopoulos I, Kikidakis D, et al. Conservative management of post-radical prostatectomy incontinence. Archivos Españoles de Urología. 2013;**66**(8):763-775

[17] Averbeck MA, Marcelissen T, Anding R, et al. How can we prevent postprostatectomy urinary incontinence by patient selection, and by preoperative, peroperative, and postoperative measures? International consultation on incontinence-research society 2018. Neurourology and Urodynamics. 2019;**38**(Suppl. 5):S119-S126. DOI: 10.1002/nau.23972

[18] Koraitim MM. The male urethral sphincter complex revisited: An anatomical concept and its physiological correlate. The Journal of Urology. 2008;**179**(5):1683-1689. DOI: 10.1016/j.juro.2008.01.010

[19] Petros PE, Woodman PJ. The integral theory of continence. International Urogynecology Journal and Pelvic Floor Dysfunction. 2008;**19**(1):35-40. DOI: 10.1007/s00192-007-0475-9

[20] Stolzenburg JU, Kallidonis P, Hicks J, et al. Effect of bladder neck preservation during endoscopic extraperitoneal radical prostatectomy on urinary continence. Urologia Internationalis. 2010;**85**(2):135-138. DOI: 10.1159/000314842

[21] Selli C, De Antoni P, Moro U, et al. Role of bladder neck preservation in urinary continence following radical retropubic prostatectomy. Scandinavian Journal of Urology and Nephrology. 2004;**38**(1):32-37. DOI: 10.1080/00365590310017280

[22] Marien TP, Lepor H. Does a nerve-sparing technique or potency affect continence after open radical retropubic prostatectomy? BJU International. 2008;**102**(11):1581-1584. DOI: 10.1111/j.1464-410X.2008.07921.x

[23] Groutz A, Blaivas JG, Chaikin DC, et al. The pathophysiology of post-radical prostatectomy incontinence: A clinical and video urodynamic study. The Journal of Urology. 2000;**163**(6):1767-1770

[24] Strasser H, Frauscher F, Helweg G, et al. Transurethral ultrasound: Evaluation of anatomy and function of the rhabdosphincter of the male urethra. The Journal of Urology. 1998;**159**(1):100-104; discussion 104-5. DOI: 10.1016/s0022-5347(01)64025-4

[25] Majoros A, Bach D, Keszthelyi A, et al. Urinary incontinence and voiding dysfunction after radical retropubic prostatectomy (prospective urodynamic study). Neurourology and Urodynamics. 2006;**25**(1):2-7. DOI: 10.1002/nau.20190

[26] Murphy DG, Costello AJ. How can the autonomic nervous system contribute to urinary continence following radical prostatectomy? A "boson-like" conundrum. European Urology. 2013;**63**(3):445-447. DOI: 10.1016/j.eururo.2012.08.031

[27] Catarin MV, Manzano GM, Nóbrega JA, et al. The role of membranous urethral afferent autonomic innervation in the continence mechanism after nerve sparing radical prostatectomy: A clinical and prospective study. The Journal of Urology. 2008;**180**(6):2527-2531. DOI: 10.1016/j.juro.2008.08.020

[28] Ozdemir MB, Eskicorapci SY, Baydar DE, et al. A cadaveric histological investigation of the prostate with three-dimensional reconstruction for better results in continence and erectile function after radical prostatectomy. Prostate Cancer and Prostatic Diseases. 2007;**10**(1):77-81. DOI: 10.1038/sj.pcan.4500917

[29] Kaye DR, Hyndman ME, Segal RL, et al. Urinary outcomes are significantly affected by nerve sparing quality during radical prostatectomy. Urology. 2013;**82**(6):1348-1353. DOI: 10.1016/j.urology.2013.06.067

[30] Sanchez-Salas R, Tourinho Barbosa R, Sivaraman A, et al. 25 - The IMPROVE trial: Surgical technique remains the most important factor associated with recovery of urinary continence after radical prostatectomy. European Urology Open Science. 2023;**48**(Supplement 1):S27. DOI: 10.1016 S2666-1683(23)00050-2

[31] Steiner MS. The puboprostatic ligament and the male urethral suspensory mechanism: An anatomic study. Urology. 1994;**44**(4):530-534. DOI: 10.1016/s0090-4295(94)80052-9

[32] Zhang C, Ding ZH, Li GX, et al. Perirectal fascia and spaces: Annular distribution pattern around the mesorectum. Diseases of the Colon and Rectum. 2010;**53**(9):1315-1322. DOI: 10.1007/DCR.0b013e3181e74525

[33] Kirschner-Hermanns R, Wein B, Niehaus S, et al. The contribution of magnetic resonance imaging of the pelvic floor to the understanding of urinary incontinence. British Journal of Urology. 1993;**72**(5 Pt 2):715-718. DOI: 10.1111/j.1464-410x.1993.tb16254.x

[34] Gosling JA, Dixon JS, Critchley HO, et al. A comparative study of the human external sphincter and periurethral levator ani muscles. British Journal of Urology. 1981;**53**(1):35-41. DOI: 10.1111/j.1464-410x.1981.tb03125.x

[35] Soljanik I, Bauer RM, Becker AJ, et al. Is a wider angle of the membranous urethra associated with incontinence after radical prostatectomy? World Journal of Urology. 2014;**32**(6):1375-1383. DOI: 10.1007/s00345-014-1241-5

[36] Tan GY, Jhaveri JK, Tewari AK. Anatomic restoration technique: A biomechanics-based approach for early continence recovery after minimally invasive radical prostatectomy. Urology. 2009;**74**(3):492-496. DOI: 10.1016/j.urology.2009.02.005

[37] Rocco F, Carmignani L, Acquati P, et al. Early continence recovery after open radical prostatectomy with restoration of the posterior aspect of the rhabdosphincter. European Urology. 2007;**52**(2):376-383. DOI: 10.1016/j.eururo.2007.01.109

[38] Nguyen MM, Kamoi K, Stein RJ, et al. Early continence outcomes of posterior musculofascial plate reconstruction during robotic and laparoscopic prostatectomy. BJU International. 2008;**101**(9):1135-1139. DOI: 10.1111/j.1464-410X.2007.07425.x

[39] Porena M, Mearini E, Mearini L, et al. Voiding dysfunction after radical retropubic prostatectomy: More than external urethral sphincter deficiency. European Urology. 2007;**52**(1):38-45. DOI: 10.1016/j.eururo.2007.03.051

[40] Matsukawa Y, Hattori R, Komatsu T, et al. De novo detrusor underactivity after laparoscopic radical prostatectomy. International Journal of Urology. 2010;**17**(7):643-648. DOI: 10.1111/j.1442-2042.2010.02529.x

[41] Lucas MG, Bosch RJ, Burkhard FC, et al. EAU guidelines on assessment and

nonsurgical management of urinary incontinence. European Urology. 2012;**62**:1130-1142. DOI: 10.1016/j.eururo.2012.08.047

[42] Averbeck MA, Woodhouse C, Comiter C, et al. Surgical treatment of post-prostatectomy stress urinary incontinence in adult men: Report from the 6th international consultation on incontinence. Neurourology and Urodynamics. 2019;**38**(1):398-406. DOI: 10.1002/nau.23845

[43] Griffiths DJ, McCracken PN, Harrison GM, et al. Relationship of fluid intake to voluntary micturition and urinary incontinence in geriatric patients. Neurourology and Urodynamics. 1993;**12**(1):1-7. DOI: 10.1002/nau.1930120102

[44] Avery K, Donovan J, Peters TJ, et al. ICIQ: A brief and robust measure for evaluating the symptoms and impact of urinary incontinence. Neurourology and Urodynamics. 2004;**23**(4):322-330. DOI: 10.1002/nau.20041

[45] Litwin MS, Hays RD, Fink A, et al. The UCLA prostate cancer index: Development, reliability, and validity of a health-related quality of life measure. Medical Care. 1998;**36**(7):1002-1012. DOI: 10.1097/00005650-199807000-00007

[46] Sacco E, Bientinesi R, Gandi C, et al. Objectively improving appropriateness of absorbent products provision to patients with urinary incontinence: The DIAPPER study. Neurourology and Urodynamics. 2018;**37**(1):485-495. DOI: 10.1002/nau.23335

[47] Sacco E, Bientinesi R, Gandi C, et al. Patient pad count is a poor measure of urinary incontinence compared with 48-h pad test: Results of a large-scale multicentre study. BJU International. 2019;**123**(5A):E69-E78. DOI: 10.1111/bju.14566

[48] Khouri RK Jr, Ortiz NM, Baumgarten AS, et al. Artificial urinary sphincter outperforms sling for moderate male stress urinary incontinence. Urology. 2020;**141**:168-172. DOI: 10.1016/j.urology.2020.03.028

[49] Karantanis E, Fynes M, Moore KH, et al. Comparison of the ICIQ-SF and 24-hour pad test with other measures for evaluating the severity of urodynamic stress incontinence. International Urogynecology Journal and Pelvic Floor Dysfunction. 2004;**15**(2):111-116; discussion 116. DOI: 10.1007/s00192-004-1123-2

[50] Bauer RM, Gozzi C, Roosen A, et al. Impact of the 'repositioning test' on postoperative outcome of retroluminar transobturator male sling implantation. Urologia Internationalis. 2013;**90**(3):334-338. DOI: 10.1159/000347123

[51] Smith WJ, VanDyke ME, Venishetty N, et al. Surgical Management of Male Stress Incontinence: Techniques, indications, and pearls for success. Research and Reports in Urology. 2023;**15**:217-232. DOI: 10.2147/RRU.S395359

[52] Barnard J, van Rij S, Westenberg AM. A Valsalva leak-point pressure of >100 cmH2O is associated with greater success in AdVance™ sling placement for the treatment of post-prostatectomy urinary incontinence. BJU International. 2014;**114**(Suppl. 1):34-37. DOI: 10.1111/bju.12791

[53] Ajay D, Kahokehr AA, Lentz AC, et al. Valsalva leak point pressure (VLPP) greater than 70 cm H2O is an indicator for sling success: A success prediction model for the male transobturator sling. International Urology and Nephrology.

2022;**54**(7):1499-1503. DOI: 10.1007/s11255-022-03222-4

[54] Han JS, Brucker BM, Demirtas A, et al. Treatment of post-prostatectomy incontinence with male slings in patients with impaired detrusor contractility on urodynamics and/or who perform Valsalva voiding. The Journal of Urology. 2011;**186**(4):1370-1375. DOI: 10.1016/j.juro.2011.05.089

[55] Trigo Rocha F, Gomes CM, Mitre AI, et al. A prospective study evaluating the efficacy of the artificial sphincter AMS 800 for the treatment of postradical prostatectomy urinary incontinence and the correlation between preoperative urodynamic and surgical outcomes. Urology. 2008;**71**(1):85-89. DOI: 10.1016/j.urology.2007.09.009

[56] Cornu JN, Melot C, Haab F. A pragmatic approach to the characterization and effective treatment of male patients with postprostatectomy incontinence. Current Opinion in Urology. 2014;**24**(6):566-570. DOI: 10.1097/MOU.0000000000000112

[57] Freitas PS, Alves AS, Correia PS, et al. Urethrocystography: A guide for urological surgery? Diagnostic and Interventional Radiology. 2023;**29**(1):9-17. DOI: 10.5152/dir.2022.21640

[58] Wolin KY, Luly J, Sutcliffe S, et al. Risk of urinary incontinence following prostatectomy: The role of physical activity and obesity. The Journal of Urology. 2010;**183**(2):629-633. DOI: 10.1016/j.juro.2009.09.082

[59] Siegel AL. Pelvic floor muscle training in males: Practical applications. Urology. 2014;**84**(1):1-7. DOI: 10.1016/j.urology.2014.03.016

[60] Tienforti D, Sacco E, Marangi F, et al. Efficacy of an assisted low-intensity programme of perioperative pelvic floor muscle training in improving the recovery of continence after radical prostatectomy: A randomized controlled trial. BJU International. 2012;**110**(7):1004-1010. DOI: 10.1111/j.1464-410X.2012.10948.x

[61] Ribeiro LH, Prota C, Gomes CM, et al. Long-term effect of early postoperative pelvic floor biofeedback on continence in men undergoing radical prostatectomy: A prospective, randomized, controlled trial. The Journal of Urology. 2010;**184**(3):1034-1039. DOI: 10.1016/j.juro.2010.05.040

[62] Goode PS, Burgio KL, Johnson TM 2nd, et al. Behavioral therapy with or without biofeedback and pelvic floor electrical stimulation for persistent postprostatectomy incontinence: A randomized controlled trial. Journal of the American Medical Association. 2011;**305**(2):151-159. DOI: 10.1001/jama.2010.1972

[63] Cardozo L, Rovner E, Wagg A, Wein A, Abrams P. Incontinence 7th Edition. Bristol UK: ICI-ICS. International Continence Society; 2023. ISBN: 978-0-9569607-4-0

[64] Berghmans B, Hendriks E, Bernards A, et al. Electrical stimulation with non-implanted electrodes for urinary incontinence in men. Cochrane Database of Systematic Reviews. 2013;**6**:CD001202. DOI: 10.1002/14651858.CD001202.pub5

[65] Radadia KD, Farber NJ, Shinder B, et al. Management of Postradical Prostatectomy Urinary Incontinence: A review. Urology. 2018;**113**:13-19. DOI: 10.1016/j.urology.2017.09.025

[66] Alan C, Eren AE, Ersay AR, et al. Efficacy of duloxetine in the early Management of Urinary Continence

after radical prostatectomy. Current Urology. 2015;**8**(1):43-48. DOI: 10.1159/000365688

[67] Kotecha P, Sahai A, Malde S. Use of duloxetine for Postprostatectomy stress urinary incontinence: A systematic review. European Urology Focus. 2021;**7**(3):618-628. DOI: 10.1016/j.euf.2020.06.007

[68] Cornu JN, Merlet B, Ciofu C, et al. Duloxetine for mild to moderate postprostatectomy incontinence: Preliminary results of a randomised, placebo-controlled trial. European Urology. 2011;**59**(1):148-154. DOI: 10.1016/j.eururo.2010.10.031

[69] Schlenker B, Gratzke C, Reich O, et al. Preliminary results on the off-label use of duloxetine for the treatment of stress incontinence after radical prostatectomy or cystectomy. European Urology. 2006;**49**(6):1075-1078. DOI: 10.1016/j.eururo.2006.01.038

[70] Collazos F, Ramos M, Qureshi A, et al. Effectiveness and tolerability of duloxetine in 2 different ethnic samples: A prospective observational cohort study. Journal of Clinical Psychopharmacology. 2013;**33**(2):254-256. DOI: 10.1097/JCP.0b013e31828567d4

[71] Fink KG, Huber J, Würnschimmel E, et al. The use of duloxetine in the treatment of male stress urinary incontinence. Wiener Medizinische Wochenschrift (1946). 2008;**158**(3-4):116-118. DOI: 10.1007/s10354-007-0494-7

[72] Filocamo MT, Li Marzi V, Del Popolo G, et al. Pharmacologic treatment in postprostatectomy stress urinary incontinence. European Urology. 2007;**51**(6):1559-1564. DOI: 10.1016/j.eururo.2006.08.005

[73] Candela L, Marra G, Tutolo M, et al. Postoperative non-surgical interventions to improve urinary continence after robot-assisted radical prostatectomy: A systematic review. Société Internationale d'Urologie Journal. 2022;**3**(2):88-100. DOI: 10.48083/DPRH8648

[74] Gravas S, Cornu JN, Gacci M, et al. European Association of Urology (EAU) Guidelines on Management of Non-Neurogenic Male Lower Urinary Tract Symptoms (LUTS), incl. Benign Prostatic Obstruction (BPO). 2022. Available from: https://uroweb.org/guidelines/management-of-non-neurogenic-male-luts [Accessed: June 2023]

[75] Sacco E, Gandi C, Marino F, et al. Artificial urinary sphincter significantly better than fixed sling for moderate post-prostatectomy stress urinary incontinence: A propensity score-matched study. BJU International. 2021;**127**(2):229-237. DOI: 10.1111/bju.15197

[76] Scott FB, Bradley WE, Timm GW. Treatment of urinary incontinence by implantable prosthetic sphincter. Urology. 1973;**1**:252-259. DOI: 10.1016/0090-4295(73)90749-8

[77] Van der Aa F, Drake MJ, Kasyan GR, et al. The artificial urinary sphincter after a quarter of a century: A critical systematic review of its use in male non-neurogenic incontinence. European Urology. 2013;**63**(4):681-689. DOI: 10.1016/j.eururo.2012.11.034

[78] Sacco E, Marino F, Gandi C, et al. Transalbugineal artificial urinary sphincter: A refined implantation technique to improve surgical outcomes. Journal of Clinical Medicine. 2023;**12**(8):3021. DOI: 10.3390/jcm12083021

[79] Wilson SK, Delk JR 2nd. Ectopic placement of AMS 800 urinary control system pressure-regulating

balloon. Urology. 2005;**65**(1):167-170. DOI: 10.1016/j.urology.2004.09.042

[80] Danforth TL, Ginsberg DA. Artificial urinary sphincter. In: Smith JA, Howards SS, Preminger GM, Dmochowski RR, editors. Hinman's Atlas of Urologic Surgery. 4th ed. Philadelphia, PA, USA: Elsevier; 2017

[81] Guralnick ML, Miller E, Toh KL, et al. Transcorporal artificial urinary sphincter cuff placement in cases requiring revision for erosion and urethral atrophy. The Journal of Urology. 2002;**167**(5):2075-2078; discussion 2079

[82] Miller D, Pekala K, Zhang X, et al. Outcomes of initial Transcorporal versus standard placement of artificial urinary sphincter in patients with prior radiation. Cureus. 2022;**14**(5):e25519. DOI: 10.7759/cureus.25519

[83] Smith PJ, Hudak SJ, Scott JF, et al. Transcorporal artificial urinary sphincter cuff placement is associated with a higher risk of postoperative urinary retention. The Canadian Journal of Urology. 2013;**20**(3):6773-6777

[84] Linder BJ, Rivera ME, Ziegelmann MJ, et al. Long-term outcomes following artificial urinary sphincter placement: An analysis of 1082 cases at Mayo Clinic. Urology. 2015;**86**(3):602-607. DOI: 10.1016/j.urology.2015.05.029

[85] Eswara JR, Chan R, Vetter JM, et al. Revision techniques after artificial urinary sphincter failure in men: Results from a multicenter study. Urology. 2015;**86**(1):176-180. DOI: 10.1016/j.urology.2015.04.023

[86] Ameli G, Weibl P, Rutkowski M, et al. A single center study to evaluate the efficacy and safety of a new adjustable artificial urinary sphincter (victo)results after follow-up>12 months. Urology. 2020;**203**(4):e731

[87] Weibl P, Hoelzel R, Rutkowski M, et al. VICTO and VICTO-plus—Novel alternative for the mangement of postprostatectomy incontinence. Early perioperative and postoperative experience. Cent European. The Journal of Urology. 2018;**71**(2):248-249. DOI: 10.5173/ceju.2018.1655

[88] Ostrowski I, Ciechan J, Sledz E, et al. Four-year follow-up on a Zephyr surgical implants 375 artificial urinary sphincter for male urinary incontinence from one urological Centre in Poland. Central European Journal of Urology. 2018;**71**(3):320-325. DOI: 10.5173/ceju.2018.1704

[89] Gozzi C, Bauer RM, Becker AJ, et al. Die funktionelle retrourethrale Schlinge. Ein Paradigmenwechsel in der Therapie der Belastungsinkontinenz nach radikaler Prostatektomie [functional retrourethral sling. A change of paradigm in the treatment of stress incontinence after radical prostatectomy]. Urologe A. 2008;**47**(9):1224-1228. German. DOI: 10.1007/s00120-008-1840-0

[90] Kaufman JJ. Urethral compression operations for the treatment of post-prostatectomy incontinence. The Journal of Urology. 1973;**110**(1):93-96. DOI: 10.1016/s0022-5347(17)60125-3

[91] Zeif H, Almallah Z. The male sling for post-radical prostatectomy urinary incontinence: Urethral compression versus urethral relocation or what is next? British Journal of Medical and Surgical Urology. 2010;**3**:134-143. DOI: 10.1016/j.bjmsu.2010.01.006

[92] Sandhu JS, Breyer B, Comiter C, et al. Incontinence after prostate treatment. AUA/SUFU guideline. Journal of

Urology. 2019;**202**:369-378. DOI: 10.1097/JU.0000000000000314

[93] Ko KJ, Kim SJ, Cho ST. Sling surgery for male urinary incontinence including post prostatectomy incontinence: A challenge to the urologist. International Neurourology Journal. 2019;**23**(3):185-194. DOI: 10.5213/inj.1938108.054

[94] Rizvi IG, Ravindra P, Pipe M, et al. The AdVance™ male sling: Does it stand the test of time? Scandinavian Journal of Urology. 2021;**55**(2):155-160. DOI: 10.1080/21681805.2021.1877342

[95] Bauer RM, Grabbert MT, Klehr B, et al. 36-month data for the AdVance XP® male sling: Results of a prospective multicentre study. BJU International. 2017;**119**(4):626-630. DOI: 10.1111/bju.13704

[96] Sacco E, Gandi C, Bientinesi R, et al. 33—Bulbospongiosus muscle-sparing AdVanceXP male sling placement: Potential benefits of a different surgical technique. Continence. 2022;**2**(Supplement 1):100074. DOI: 10.1016/j.cont.2022.100074

[97] Meisterhofer K, Herzog S, Strini KA, et al. Male slings for Postprostatectomy incontinence: A systematic review and meta-analysis. European Urology Focus. 2020;**6**(3):575-592. DOI: 10.1016/j.euf.2019.01.008

[98] Constable L, Abrams P, Cooper D, et al. Synthetic sling or artificial urinary sphincter for men with urodynamic stress incontinence after prostate surgery: The MASTER non-inferiority RCT. Health Technology Assessment. 2022;**26**(36):1-152. DOI: 10.3310/TBFZ0277

[99] Davies TO, Bepple JL, McCammon KA. Urodynamic changes and initial results of the AdVance male sling. Urology. 2009;**74**(2):354-357. DOI: 10.1016/j.urology.2008.12.082

[100] Bauer RM, Bastian PJ, Gozzi C, et al. Postprostatectomy incontinence: All about diagnosis and management. European Urology. 2009;**55**(2):322-333. DOI: 10.1016/j.eururo.2008.10.029

[101] Bole R, Hebert KJ, Gottlich HC, et al. Narrative review of male urethral sling for post-prostatectomy stress incontinence: Sling type, patient selection, and clinical applications. Translational Andrology and Urology. 2021;**10**(6):2682-2694. DOI: 10.21037/tau-20-1459

[102] Munier P, Nicolas M, Tricard T, et al. What if artificial urinary sphincter is not possible? Feasibility and effectiveness of ProACT for patients with persistent stress urinary incontinence after radical prostatectomy treated by sling. Neurourology and Urodynamics. 2020;**39**(5):1417-1422. DOI: 10.1002/nau.24355

[103] Ha YS, Yoo ES. Artificial urinary sphincter for Postradical prostatectomy urinary incontinence—Is it the best option? International Neurourology Journal. 2019;**23**(4):265-276. DOI: 10.5213/inj.1938210.105

[104] Lebret T, Cour F, Benchetrit J, et al. Treatment of postprostatectomy stress urinary incontinence using a minimally invasive adjustable continence balloon device, ProACT: Results of a preliminary, multicenter, pilot study. Urology. 2008;**71**(2):256-260. DOI: 10.1016/j.urology.2007.08.062

[105] Mühlstädt S, Angulo JC, Mohammed N, et al. Complications of the urinary incontinence system ATOMS: Description of risk factors and how to prevent these pitfalls. World Journal of Urology. 2020;**38**(7):1795-1803. DOI: 10.1007/s00345-019-02962-w

[106] Toia B, Gresty H, Pakzad M, et al. Bulking for stress urinary incontinence in men: A systematic review. Neurourology and Urodynamics. 2019;**38**(7):1804-1811. DOI: 10.1002/nau.24102

[107] Chong JT, Simma-Chiang V. A historical perspective andevolution of the treatment of male urinary incontinence. Neurourology and Urodynamics. 2018;**37**(3):1169-1175

[108] Salciccia S, Viscuso P, Bevilacqua G, et al. Comparison of different invasive devices for the treatment of urinary incontinence after radical prostatectomy. Advances in Urology. 2022;**2022**:8736249. DOI: 10.1155/2022/8736249

Section 5

Improving the Hospital Environment

Chapter 9

The Environmental Impact on Advanced Midwives from Underutilization in Tertiary Hospital

Mbulaheni Rhona Luphai

Abstract

Advanced midwifery practice is an autonomous status that is developed during midwifery training and practices. Advanced midwives in their practice are expected to take full responsibility when it comes to patients under their care. However, in tertiary hospitals, all the care given to maternity patients yields grey area which needs responsibility sharing between the midwives and other multidisciplinary team members like obstetric doctors and paediatric doctors. The tertiary environment is overclouded by medical-dependent practices which is widened by the communication gap between the multidisciplinary teams. Lack of professional communication in tertiary hospitals' work environment when it comes to sharing of accountability pushes the midwives to their cocoon shells which make them lose their patient advocacy role, knowledge, and skills. Based on the environmental expectations, set ups and practices, patients end up receiving compromised maternity care which open doors to major malpractices and complications like unnecessary loss of lives and litigations. In the presence of malpractices, there is always a tendency of the multidisciplinary team members blaming each other and mostly the blamed professionals are the midwives which strains the environmental professional relationships.

Keywords: advanced midwife, tertiary hospital, teamwork, multidisciplinary team, professional communication, and underutilization

1. Introduction

Tertiary work environment in the maternal healthcare service is the key role player in the psychological aspects of the multidisciplinary team members which include midwives. In some developing countries the staffing norms in tertiary hospitals is mandated by the country's maternity guidelines which require midwives with extra qualifications of advanced midwife and neonatal science to be allocated in substantial number to manage the high-risk type of patients in those level of care situation. However, due to shortage of advanced midwives in most countries, makes it impossible to meet that prescribed mandate of accumulating the required number of that category of staff which is also complicated by the high volume of patients in such a high level of care. The high volume of patients with a shortage of staff makes the tertiary hospital environment to be psychologically stressful for healthcare providers. A psychologically stable-minded midwife's performance is depicted by the decisions taken in the management of patient care process communication with other members of the multidisciplinary team, pregnant, birthing, and post-birth women. The psychologically stable-minded midwives provide holistic care with passion, respect, dignity, and with confident to maternity patients under their care. Tertiary maternity patients are significantly unstable patients with significantly demanding high levels of care.

Tertiary maternity patients are referred patients with obstetric emergencies from lower levels of care areas which can either be a primary health care clinic, midwifery obstetric unit (MOU), district hospitals, and regional hospitals. The common indicators for obstetric emergency referrals include preterm labour; pregnancy-induced hypertension; fatal distress; previous caesarean section; malpresentation; cord prolapse, shoulder dystocia, placenta praevia, amniotic fluid embolism poor progress in labour, infections. Obstetric emergency patients are stressful to manage and necessitate a healthy environment which needs the full involvement of all professionals in the rendering of care [1]. Obstetric emergencies are the main causes of the unnecessary preventable or unpreventable loss of the mother or loss of the baby, or loss of which are stressful situation for the midwives looking after the patient. In that stressful environment, advanced midwives are keen, dedicated, and committed to support maternity women even if there are challenges like a language barrier between them and the patient, with system lack of midwife support as the maternity systems lack accessible interpretation services to support women with language needs which make midwives go through stressful experiences of falling through the net as it came out as one of the findings of study conducted by midwives [2]. The status of the type of patients who are managed in tertiary hospitals is at considerable risk of prolonged hospitalisation, complications related to their conditions, and mother or baby, or both losing lives. Prolonged patient hospitalisation creates a special bonding between patients and the midwives which is very traumatic psychologically to the midwives in situation where the outcome of care does not go as planned like in the development of severe complications and loss of life. However, in such stressful situations, advanced midwives are restricted to fully utilise their knowledge and skills. Most psychological stress is contributed by not being given full opportunity to be involved in the planning of maternity patient care which leads to lack of full utilisation of own midwifery professional knowledge and skills. Lack or no utilisation of own professional knowledge and skills in overcrowded tertiary hospitals with a lack of midwife-patient ratio, prolonged working hours, shortage of midwives, and experiences over number of each encounters with patients causes psychological stress to midwives. The underutilization of the midwifery knowledge and skills was affirmed by the study conducted in the four tertiary hospitals, where findings affirmed that the advanced midwives' skills and knowledge are not fully utilised [3]. There are several contributory factors that lead to underutilization of advanced midwives in tertiary hospitals. Lack of teamwork and lack of respect within the multidisciplinary team in tertiary obstetric working environment is the contributory factor to the midwife's psychological stresses. Studies confirm that obstetricians do recognise advanced midwives' qualifications and competencies but still see midwives as professionals who lack the skills and competency to be independent practitioners who can manage, intervene, and make confident decisions in each obstetric situation [4]. The undermining attitudes of doctors were exposed in the primary healthcare setting in the upscaling of midwives' skills to ordering medications when most doctors working in maternity hospitals were more sceptical and believing that midwives were not equipped enough to order medications. The findings further suggested that as midwives they are being able to re-order medications that were prescribed by doctors first [5]. The undermining and underutilization of the possessed knowledge and skills obtained through the midwifery professional registration body in the tertiary hospitals turn the environment to be toxic causing stress to midwives. Advanced midwifery training puts the midwives into the autonomous practitioner's status.

2. Underutilization of the advanced midwives who are autonomous practitioners

Advanced midwives as one of the advanced nursing qualifications globally are the midwives who are trained to achieve elevated levels of universal quality maternal care. The level and utilisation of the achieved knowledge and skill by the advanced midwife is globally according to the expectations of practice from the specific country that is training the advanced nurse practitioner. Advanced midwives go through a higher level of training which gives them the elevated level of knowledge and skills to practice midwifery care with attributes such as effective people skills, thoughtfulness, self-reliance, clarity of thoughts, self-evaluation, and self-confidence with the ability to reflect and analyse observations and care given to pregnant women, birthing women and their babies, and post-births women and their families [6]. In the process of advanced midwifery training, it is mandatory that the achievement of the success in training are measured and assessed through competencies in direct patient care, collaboration with multidisciplinary team, consultation in managing elevated risk conditions, and leadership skills. Competences acquired include skilfulness in managing obstetric complications like shoulder dystocia, breech delivery, resuscitations of newborns, vacuum extractions, and interpretations of statistics in maternity healthcare services. The elevated level of competency, knowledge, and skills acquired during the advanced midwives training prepares them to play the pivotal role of being the backbone of the maternal healthcare services. However, there are barriers to using all this learned because there is lack of clear job description for the advanced midwives in the tertiary hospital setting to enable them to utilise them their acquired knowledge and skills. The possession of the advanced skills and advanced knowledge by advanced midwives from their training, put them in the crucial point of care as an autonomous practitioner who is equipped to vigilantly stays with the patient in the prolonged hours of duty shifts. For midwives to fully fulfil their duties, clear policies of dealing with the four crucial areas of care need to be developed or dealt with in the tertiary hospitals which will allow midwives to fully function according to their scope of practice. Lack of policies directing the full functioning of the advanced midwives in the crucial areas of care identified by the midwives are the leading course of midwives challenges in tertiary hospitals in performing professional duties in the following four areas: full function to quality patient care, full contribution to teaching, dealing with managerial roles, and dealing with the admission of patients [3]. The impact of underutilization of the possessed knowledge and skills are seen in the contribution of quality patient care, contribution in teaching, dealing with managerial roles, and dealing with the admission of patients which are shown in **Figure 1**.

2.1 Underutilization impact in the contribution of quality patient care

Midwives are professional practitioners who are expected to fully contribute to patient care by being with the patient continuously in the patient's stay in the hospital.

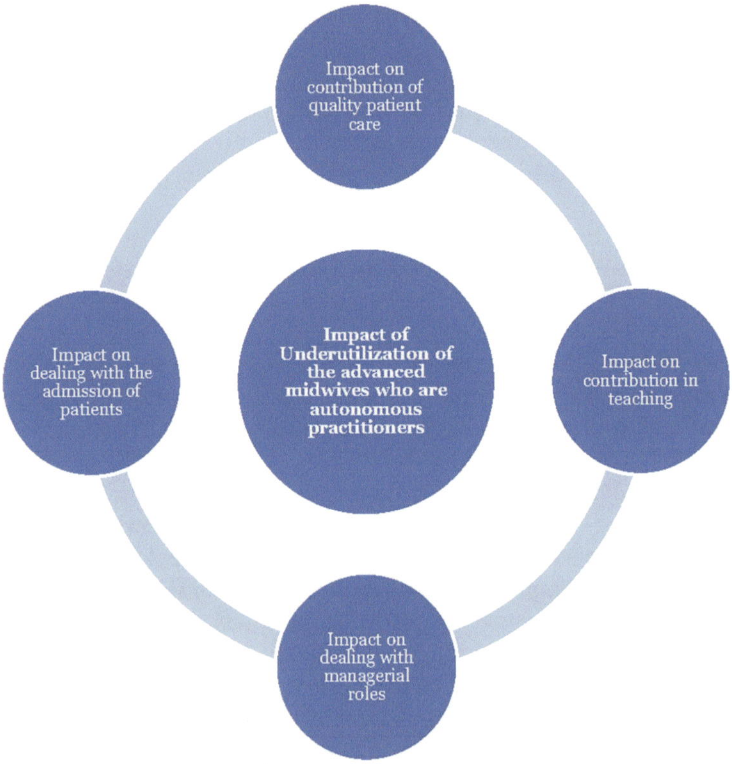

Figure 1.
Impact of underutilization of the advanced midwives who are autonomous practitioners.

The major expectations in that giving of care include using the full role in rendering patient clinical care, patient advocacy, leadership in maternity care, and role modelling partnership with the multidisciplinary team. However, there are stressful hindrances in using all these expectations due to a lack of proper clarification of the advanced midwives in tertiary hospital environments in countries. The stressful environmental challenges which are available in the maternity areas and affecting the maternal healthcare services births experiences were even picked up by the international federations of midwives, gynaecologists, and obstetricians [7]. The International Confederation of the Midwives (ICM) and the Federation of International Gynaecological Obstetrics (FIGO) has greater support of close teamwork and recognition of the interdisciplinary collaboration between obstetricians, other healthcare providers, and midwives in support of the woman in labour and partner, coming baby, and the family at large. In addition to that recognition, FIGO and ICM are working towards up-to-date guidelines which are midwifery enabling to the working environments.

In the rendering of care, midwives are to take full responsibility for the monitoring of the quality care which is received by the patients including the evaluation of the patient condition and mostly with the condition of the coming baby. To perform that watching and evaluating a function, the midwife needs to practice the skill to remain knowledgeable and skilful. It is unfortunate for the advanced midwives in tertiary hospitals as the procedures are performed by the medical doctors due to the conditions of the patients who are hospitalised. The main challenge is that when it comes to planning care for the same patients the midwives are catering, when it comes to the involvement in decision making there is lack of midwives' involvement in the multidisciplinary team. Lack of midwives' involvement in planning and decision-making in the care given to patients pushes the midwives to their cocoon space which leads to defensive midwifery practice which does not improve the maternal healthcare services. The defensive midwifery practice is one of just conducting doctors' orders and prescriptions without evaluation and documenting own performance which is psychologically stressful to the midwives. Tertiary hospitals are full of medical doctors in training who still need guidance in their maternity practices. However, due to a lack of structured communication and clear role descriptions of the advanced midwives, even the training obstetricians are taking decisions without discussing the patient with the midwives. Teamwork and full use of all team members is the key to saving patients' lives which is the main aims of tertiary hospital care. However, there are studies which exposed that the functionality of the multidisciplinary team lacks full involvement of the other team members like advanced midwives which leads to the underutilization of their knowledge and skills. The main purpose of multidisciplinary care is to enable all team members to consensually reach an agreement on the type of care to be provided to the patients.

Midwives do understand that in tertiary hospitals the responsibility of care has grey area for sharing, and that doctors take full responsibility. However, having been equipped with knowledge and skills which is not practiced make them a scapegoat for the malpractices in the tertiary hospitals as one of the midwives' roles is to take a lead in advocating for the pregnant women, unborn babies, and the newborns under their care in the multidisciplinary team. Midwives are more productive in the rendering of care in the work environment which enables them to serve with a reflection of their personal and professional philosophies as midwives. The midwife's professional philosophy is shown when they are collaborating with colleagues who have the descent work ethics, when they practice their passion of advocating for pregnant women, babies, and family members under their care. In the healthcare system, nurses and midwives are the centre in the provision of the autonomous care which reflect in the collaboration of the multidisciplinary groups of community in different settings of care. The continuous stay of the midwives with the maternity patients requires them to be spokespersons or advocators for those who cannot talk like newborns, terribly ill women, the scared and the shy patients who cannot talk for themselves in the multidisciplinary team care. The advocacy role of the nurse and the midwife are the key roles in the management of the maternal healthcare system [8]. In tertiary hospitals midwife's advocacy role if fully utilised, can save patients' lives, and prevent unnecessary complications which lead to litigations. In case of loss of life and complications there is always increased level of self-blame to midwives as they are equipped with knowledge and skills for caring and for advocacy in their midwifery training. The contributory factor of blocked advocacy is being belittled by medical doctors, lack of respect from doctors when it comes to taking midwives advice and involving midwives in planning patient's care [3]. Lack of the use of the multidisciplinary team knowledge and skill in supplying quality care contributes to midwives' psychological stresses in tertiary healthcare services.

2.2 Underutilization impact in teaching contributions

Teaching function is one of the midwives' professional mandates. Tertiary hospitals are full of different health professional students which include medical doctors (registrars) and nurses. Knowledge sharing is a way of strengthening the rendering of quality care as skills and knowledge are shared within diverse levels of the multidisciplinary teams.

The advanced midwives are proud in sharing their skills of effective continuity of care, diagnostic accuracy, reduction of mortality rate by early detection of complications, leading the innovative service delivery, including the provision of care, which is safe and satisfactory to patients to patients. There are hinderances in the work environment which makes it difficult for knowledge sharing. Lack of human and material resources are mostly the major obstacles that prevent the smooth running of the teaching contribution part. Knowledge and skills are easily shared through the demonstration of expected quality care in the work environment. Lack of equipment contribute to sharing of skills which compromises patient care. There is a distinct lack of essential resources like delivery packs, sanitary pads, and suturing materials in the birthing units which forces midwives to compromise patient care. Through teaching the midwives are encouraged to study to adjust and cope with the different innovations of care. There are researchers who recommend the improvement of quality care and clinical education in maternal healthcare globally through the introduction of skilful midwives in clinical sites at the tertiary-levels of care hospitals with the enormous number of students [9].

Midwives lose their skills and Knowledge by working with enormous number of patients without the necessary equipment and that course stress as wrong equipment's are used for improvising the proper tools of traits. Teaching of junior staff stimulates midwives to more reading, to be innovative, and to be up to date with all clinical care needed for critically ill patients. Midwives' job satisfaction comes from providing care that is acceptable and can easily be shared with other health professionals in multidisciplinary teams. A shortage of staff with the influx of patients makes the tertiary environment impossible for the scheduled teachings by the midwives. Sharing and provision of quality patient care to women and their families are rated high in safe midwifery practices [10].

Medical and nursing students are distributed to the maternity units to reinforce and practice the skills which have been shown to them at the skills lab in nursing colleges and universities. Lack of the essential tools of traits fails the midwives' teachings and can also lead to litigations which midwives fear. Demonstrating care to medical and nursing students with improvised tools of traits reflects the incapability of keeping professional legacy, hence midwives feel discouraged to teach as students will refer to them as not teaching according to the norms and standards of the universities and colleges. Patient care without sharing knowledge and skills affects the midwives psychologically as it reduces the knowledge, skills, and confidence in midwifery practice.

2.3 Underutilization impact in dealing with managerial issues

Managerial issues are more challenging to manage in tertiary hospitals as they deviate midwives' attention from holistic patient care. The main managerial issues which are a challenge are dealing with both human resource and non-human resource issues. Managerial challenges are depicted by incomplete documentation of the care rendered as the undocumented information in maternal healthcare services reflects the unprovided patient care. The shortage of obstetricians and midwives is a global challenge which affects patient care in all levels of care in maternity healthcare services. Globally the midwives outnumber the obstetrician's number which forces midwives to perform the obstetrician's duty in case of emergencies when doctors are busy with obstetric emergency cases in theatre or in the wards [11]. However, advanced midwives are faced with challenges of the unspecified job descriptions in the upset of the doctors in the identifiable grey areas of procedures that can be performed by the doctors or the midwives. In the case of loss of life or complication, the blame will always be shifted to the midwives as they are the first contact with patients and continue monitoring the patient throughout the patient stay in the hospital. Midwives do render holistic care to maternity patients, but with a high influx of patients, midwives sometimes end up with challenges of lack of time to make clear documentation of the rendered care.

Most challenges are caused by the shortage as there is always a gap in unrendered care as there are not enough midwives who can cater for the high volume of patients in tertiary hospitals. The high volume of patients is from the non-stipulated global midwife-patient ratio in tertiary hospitals. There is also an identified lack of clinical care and support in clinical practice from nursing leadership to the healthcare providers. Midwives also need support and mentorship from leadership in the management of complicated patient care. In the current technological era where patients get more information on internet, midwives need more support from senior managers and researchers to give them the courage to implement the new birthing positions and pain relief methods. Midwives suggest on the additional midwives in the clinical areas and to be trained in different skills as a way of showing support on their midwifery practices. Lack of or minimal support and mentoring from leadership in maternal healthcare services contribute to substandard care as midwives are scared to implement the acquired skills as in case of complications, they will not be supported by the nursing managers without being blamed for practicing doctors' skills in tertiary hospitals. Hence advanced midwives end up performing routine care which does not stimulate their thinking capacity, and compromises patient care in tertiary hospitals. Lack of or poor trust among midwives, obstetricians, paediatricians, and hospital leadership increases the stress level in the tertiary maternal healthcare environment. Staffing of the maternal health services affect the care rendered to women, babies, and their families in a negative way as it causes adverse effects in their lives. Shortage of staff has been observed and identified by FIGO's Safe Motherhood and Newborn Health Committee which came up with the proposal of having standards staffing policy setting which starts from the labour wards, and the staffing to take into consideration the volume of deliveries in the area, professional skill mix among the midwives and the obstetricians. The same committee also stressed the issue of the shift leader as the key role player in the management of shortage [12].

In that environment with gross shortages of obstetricians, paediatricians, and midwives, there is also a big challenge of non-human resource. Tools of traits are also a big challenge to maternity healthcare providers. There shortage of suitable machines for monitoring women in labour, including birthing materials. Midwives do improvise to save lives and those are the things which make them fall through the net as it increases sepsis in the maternal healthcare services. Poor or lack of patient referral systems in the countries which lead to low-risk cases landing in tertiary hospitals.

2.4 Underutilization impact in dealing with admission of patients

Advanced midwives are mandated to screen and manage maternity patients at the lower levels of care like MOU and primary healthcare services. However, due to a lack of proper coordination of maternal healthcare services, midwives find themselves managing the unbooked and self-referrals in the tertiary hospitals. The main challenge with the unbooked patients is that they miss the opportunity to be screened and managed for complications during antenatal period. Hence, they usually come in tertiary hospitals with complications which exposes them to losing their unborn babies or losing their lives. Sometimes complications do happen in the process of transferring patients between the primary healthcare services and the tertiary hospitals as the transport for transferring patients do delay or not equipped with tools of traits or adequately trained staff for managing complications. Loss of life in such circumstances causes a lot of psychological stress to healthcare providers.

3. Conclusions

This chapter highlighted the environmental impact on from the underutilization of the advanced midwives in tertiary hospitals. The discussion was underpinned by the midwife's autonomous status in the provision of care in the maternal healthcare system. The impacts were elaborated in contribution of quality care, contribution in teaching, contribution in dealing with managerial challenges, and dealing with admission of patients.

Acknowledgements

I will like to thank the almighty God who gave me strength and good health in the writing of this chapter.

There was no funding from any institution.

Conflict of interest

The author declares no conflict of interest.

Definition list

Acronyms	full meaning
MOU	midwifery obstetric unit
ICM	International Congress of Midwives
FIGO	Federation of International Gynaecologists and Obstetricians

Author details

Mbulaheni Rhona Luphai
Rahima Moosa Mother and Child Hospital, Johannesburg, Gauteng Province, South Africa

*Address all correspondence to: luphaimr@yahoo.co.uk

References

[1] Mashamba EK, Ramavhoya IT. The stress of the midwife: Experiences of advanced midwives working in obstetric emergency units in Johannesburg, South Africa. African Journal of Reproductive Health. 2021;**25**(5):93-104

[2] Bridle L, Bassett S, Silverio SA. "We couldn't talk to her": A qualitative exploration of the experiences of UK midwives when navigating women's care without language. International Journal of Human Rights in Healthcare. 2021;**14**(4):359-373

[3] Luphai MR. The role of advanced midwives regarding maternity care in tertiary hospitals in Gauteng [Master's dissertation], University of Pretoria

[4] De la Fuente-Solana EI, Suleiman-Martos N, Pradas-Hernandez L, Gomez-Urquiza JL, Canadas-De la Fuente GA, Albendín-García L. Prevalence, related factors, and levels of burnout syndrome among nurses working in gynaecology and obstetrics services: A systematic review and meta-analysis. International Journal of Environmental Research and Public Health. 2019;**16**(14):2585

[5] Zarzeka A, Panczyk M, Belowska J, Mazur N, Lourido BP, Gotlib J. Nurse prescribing: Attitudes of medical doctors towards expanding professional competencies of nurses and midwives. JPMA. The Journal of the Pakistan Medical Association. 2019;**69**(8):1199-1204

[6] Heinen M, van Oostveen C, Peters J, Vermeulen H, Huis A. An integrative review of leadership competencies and attributes in advanced nursing practice. Journal of Advanced Nursing. 2019;**75**(11):2378-2392

[7] Begum F, Beyeza J, Burke T, Evans C, Hanson C, Lalonde A, et al. FIGO and the International Confederation of Midwives endorse WHO guidelines on prevention and treatment of postpartum hemorrhage. International Journal of Gynaecology and Obstetrics. 2022;**158**(Suppl. 1):6

[8] Al-Harahsheh S, White D, Ali AM, Schnurman D, El Araybi C, Al-Mutawa MN. Nursing and Midwifery Workforce Development. Qatar: World Innovation Summit for Health and Qatar Foundation, Policy Briefing; 2020

[9] Rosanne R, Fitzpatrick JJ, Masick K. Clinical Nurses' perceptions of authentic nurse leadership and healthy work environment. JONA: The Journal of Nursing Administration. 2020;**50**(9):489-494. DOI: 10.1097/NNA.0000000000000921

[10] Matthews R, Hyde R, Llewelyn F, Shafiei T, Newton M, Forster DA. Factors associated with midwives' job satisfaction and experience of work: A cross-sectional survey of midwives in a tertiary maternity hospital in Melbourne, Australia. Women and Birth. 2022;**35**(2):e153-e162

[11] Tikkanen R, Gunja MZ, FitzGerald M, Zephyrin L. Maternal mortality and maternity care in the United States compared to 10 other developed countries. The Commonwealth Fund. 2020;**10**:22

[12] Stones W, Visser GH, Theron G, FIGO Safe Motherhood, Newborn Health Committee, Di Renzo GC, et al. FIGO statement: Staffing requirements for delivery care, with special reference to low-and middle-income countries. International Journal of Gynecology & Obstetrics. 2019;**146**(1):3-7